Free DVD 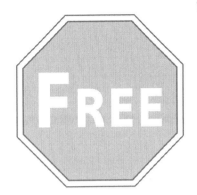 **Free DVD**

Essential Test Tips DVD from Trivium Test Prep

Dear Customer,

Thank you for purchasing from Trivium Test Prep! Whether you're looking to join the military, get into college, or advance your career, we're honored to be a part of your journey.

To show our appreciation (and to help you relieve a little of that test-prep stress), we're offering a **FREE CSCS®** *Essential Test Tips DVD* by Trivium Test Prep. Our DVD includes 35 test preparation strategies that will help keep you calm and collected before and during your big exam. All we ask is that you email us your feedback and describe your experience with our product. Amazing, awful, or just so-so: we want to hear what you have to say!

To receive your **FREE CSCS®** *Essential Test Tips DVD*, please email us at 5star@ triviumtestprep.com. Include "Free 5 Star" in the subject line and the following information in your email:

1. The title of the product you purchased.

2. Your rating from 1 – 5 (with 5 being the best).

3. Your feedback about the product, including how our materials helped you meet your goals and ways in which we can improve our products.

4. Your full name and shipping address so we can send your **FREE CSCS®** *Essential Test Tips DVD*.

If you have any questions or concerns please feel free to contact us directly at 5star@triviumtestprep.com.

Thank you, and good luck with your studies!

CSCS PRACTICE QUESTIONS TEST PREP BOOK 2021-2022

Exam Review with over 400 Practice Questions for the Certified Strength and Conditioning Test

E. M. Falgout

About the Authors

Beth Lazarou just celebrated her sixth year as a National Academy of Sports Medicine (NASM)-certified personal trainer. She is also a certified Group Fitness Instructor through the American Council on Exercise (ACE), a NASM Fitness Nutrition Specialist, and a NASM Corrective Exercise Specialist. In addition, Beth holds a Kettlebell Instruction Certification through the American Sports and Fitness Association. She specializes in social, HIIT, kettlebell, and functional fitness. Currently, Beth is attending Arizona State University's online program, pursuing a BS in Health Science.

Keith Lee Schuchardt received a BS in Exercise Science: Fitness Specialist from West Chester University of Pennsylvania. He went on to obtain an MS in Exercise Science: Health Promotion and Rehabilitation Science from California University of Pennsylvania. Keith has been certified through the National Strength and Conditioning Association (NSCA) as a Certified Strength and Conditioning Specialist, the National Academy of Sports Medicine (NASM) as a Corrective Exercise Specialist, and the American College of Sports Medicine (ACSM) as a Certified Exercise Physiologist. For over a decade, he has worked as a personal trainer in both corporate and private settings, as well as a strength and conditioning coach for professional and collegiate athletes. He is currently pursuing a Doctorate in Physical Therapy at A.T. Still University.

TABLE OF CONTENTS

INTRODUCTION

What is a Personal Trainer?

The world of personal training is vast and growing in many ways. A personal trainer is an educated exercise professional who possesses the knowledge and skill set to create and instruct others in various fitness-related settings. Personal trainers must strive to achieve a base of knowledge and to acquire the skills to properly design and implement research-based training programs that are safe and effective for their clientele. It is up to the certified personal trainer to ensure the client receives the highest quality training experience through appropriate goal setting, needs analysis, exercise prescriptions, and health and fitness education. Additionally, it is the certified personal trainer's responsibility to develop and employ these methods within his or her scope of practice. There are a variety of different career paths a certified personal trainer can pursue based on his or her interests and abilities.

Personal trainers can be productive in many different settings and businesses. The most common settings in which personal trainers work are the large, well-known gym chains and smaller, privately owned fitness centers that are common in the United States. These facilities are generally open to hiring newly trained, certified fitness professionals and are a good starting point for anyone looking to advance within a specific company.

However, there are a number of other settings in which certified personal trainers can utilize their health and fitness knowledge. For example, personal trainers can work in clinical settings, corporate training, in-home private settings, sports camps, and more. Working in a clinical setting as a personal trainer often involves administering exercise stress tests with a team supervised by a physician or medical practitioner. Corporate trainers tend to work at the private fitness centers of corporations in an office building. Some clientele prefer a more personalized workout within the privacy of their own home; the certified personal trainer will travel to the client's house with his or her equipment. Depending on the fitness professional's background, it may be preferable to work as a sports-specific strength and conditioning coach. There are many career paths available, but one key component of the personal training world is the certification.

Getting Certified

BENEFITS OF CERTIFICATION

Earning a certification through a nationally recognized fitness organization is one of the most important accomplishments for a fitness professional aiming to further his or her career. Certification is important for several reasons. First, fitness certifications require the acquisition of a substantial amount of valuable expertise and knowledge to pass the examination. Second, maintenance of most certifications requires continuing education through conventions, seminars, or other educational opportunities, so professionals keep their knowledge current and stay abreast of trends in the field. Finally, certification through major organizations demonstrates credibility to peers and clientele. The examination process requires adequate preparation to ensure successful candidates become personal trainers.

Fitness certification exams test individuals on a wide variety of exercise-science-based concepts. The concepts tested include, but are not limited to: exercise physiology, biomechanics, exercise psychology, anatomy and physiology, exercise prescription and program design, fitness facility organization and management, fitness programs for various populations, and more. Various fitness organizations provide test preparation materials such as study guides, review books, and practice tests that provide individuals with an idea of what they should expect on the exam. Fitness professionals seeking to become certified must prepare themselves for the exam by studying and being able to apply the knowledge in the materials. The certification exams are intentionally difficult in order to adequately prepare the candidates to work as competent professionals in the field of exercise science. This ensures the certified personal trainer will provide clients with safe and effective fitness programs.

Maintaining a fitness certification through the major organizations requires continued educational pursuits among the various topics in exercise science. This can be achieved through many avenues such as fitness conventions, web seminars, informational sessions with accompanying tests, and additional certifications. The purpose of continuing education credits for certifications is to ensure that the certified personal trainer maintains current knowledge and relevant expertise. Ever-improving scientific testing protocols, procedures, and equipment optimize the data that fitness professionals use to create ideal programs for clients. Studying the most up-to-date material ensures that the client is provided the most efficient method for obtaining their goals, but it is up to the trainer to guide them in the correct direction.

Credibility among trainers is ensured through the aforementioned certification process. Clientele and employers who are seeking the most qualified candidate can be assured they have a professional trainer by the certification the trainer holds. Based on the strenuous testing protocol and ongoing education requirements, certification makes it easier to determine whether a trainer is ready for a gig. High-profile employers will often require elite certifications of their training staff. For instance, professional sports teams often insist on a specific certification before considering an applicant. This requirement is often common at the collegiate level of fitness professionals as well. It shows the employers that the trainer has taken the time to understand the information relevant to providing the most effective program for their athletes.

It is highly important for individuals seeking any employment in the fitness industry to acquire certification through the major exercise organizations. The rigorous testing protocols require fitness professionals to achieve significant expertise in a variety of topics, which enhances their ability to create effective exercise programs. The major fitness organizations ensure fitness professionals keep their knowledge and expertise current. Certification supplies the employer and clients with an understanding of a fitness professional's level of credibility and competency in the field. In preparation for this great achievement, the fitness professional must first select which certification best fits his or her goals.

The following list provides information on some of the advantages and disadvantages for various major fitness certifications:

American Council on Exercise (ACE) Certification

Advantages: The ACE certifications undergo accreditation through the National Commission for Certifying Agencies (NCCA), which ensures a program's certifications are evaluated for high-quality outcomes for their professionals. There are a variety of different certification specializations that can be obtained, which provides fitness professionals with different fields of expertise to study. ACE has an agreement for guaranteed interviews with several major fitness clubs that are found throughout the United States, enhancing the ability to find potential jobs. ACE certifications do not require a college-level degree to sit for the exam. All research utilized to develop the study material is scientifically evidence-based to ensure its effectiveness.

Disadvantages: The study materials and test can be expensive, totaling over $600 for the Personal Trainers Certification alone without specializations. Higher-profile training jobs, such as professional and collegiate strength coaches, typically require certification through other organizations such as ACSM or NSCA®.

National Academy of Sports Medicine (NASM) Certification

Advantages: The NASM certifications are also accredited through the NCCA like ACE, ensuring credibility. NASM certifications also do not require a bachelor's degree to sit for examination. NASM offers a money-back guarantee in finding employment in the field within ninety days. The certification exams are difficult, but the material effectively prepares candidates for the test if studied adequately. There are a variety of different specializations to choose from, including corrective exercise, sports performance, youth training, and more. Many colleges and universities have partnered with NASM to supply certifications through classes offered at the schools.

Disadvantages: The study materials and exams are also expensive, ranging from $699 to $1,299 depending on what program is selected. The certifications do not require continuing education to maintain certification, which could potentially cause information to become obsolete.

National Strength and Conditioning Association® (NSCA®)—Certified Strength and Conditioning Specialist® (CSCS®)

Advantages: The NSCA® is accredited through the NCCA® like the previous two certifying organizations. The NSCA®—Certified Strength and Conditioning Specialist® exam is very well known nationally and with professional athletic organizations as one of the top fitness certifications. The CSCS® certification is specifically designed for preparing exercise programs for athletes and improving sports performance. Another advantage is that there are numerous study sources for the exam, including a textbook, practice exams, online and classroom clinics, and test prep materials. Also, becoming a member of the organization reduces the cost of the exam itself, and the exam is slightly cheaper than the aforementioned certifications. The textbook is thorough and excellent preparation for the exam.

Disadvantages: The NSCA®—CSCS® certification exam is difficult and contains a large amount of information and requires a lot of preparation time. Furthermore, this specific certification requires that candidates either be currently enrolled as a senior or hold a bachelor's degree in exercise science. Finally, the study materials can become pricey if more than a textbook is required.

American College of Sports Medicine (ACSM) Certification

Advantages: Like the aforementioned certifications, the ACSM certifications are accredited through the NCCA. Also, like the NSCA®, the ACSM is a highly recognized certifying fitness organization. There are multiple certifications available for those with backgrounds in exercise science (e.g., ACSM—Certified Exercise Physiologist) and those without (e.g., ACSM—Certified Personal Trainer). These certifications are designed to adequately prepare the fitness professional for exercise program design for general and special populations. The certification is excellent at teaching how to manage and stratify risks with new clientele. There are various modes of test preparation supplies similar to that of the NSCA®.

Disadvantages: Some ACSM exams require a bachelor's degree in exercise science or a related field. They have a high degree of difficulty and the preparation materials and services can be expensive. Furthermore, employers may prefer other certifications depending on the type of clientele they work with. For example, although the ACSM is considered as a gold standard in fitness, professional athletic teams may seek NSCA®—CSCS® certified trainers because they specialize in sports performance.

It is in the best interest of the fitness professional to do as much research on the various certifications as possible. This includes researching the type of environment in which the fitness professional wants to advance their career. Selecting the right certification for a specified career path in fitness can help to save a lot of money and time in the long run. It may be necessary to look into specific employers to determine which type of training certification will improve the chances for success. Additionally, researching the testing procedures and requirements will help educate the fitness professional on the level of commitment required to become a certified trainer.

National Strength and Conditioning Association® (NSCA®)—Certified Strength and Conditioning Specialist® (CSCS®)

The **National Strength and Conditioning Association®** (**NSCA®**) is one of the oldest accredited certifying fitness organizations dedicated to improving the health and fitness industry. The organization formed in 1978 as a convention for strength coaches throughout the country and has expanded to one of the leading organizations in fitness. The NSCA® has a solid foundation in exercise for improved sports performance and fitness and has developed additional certifications in tactical strength and conditioning and fitness for special populations. Current certifications include the Certified Strength and Conditioning Specialist® (CSCS®), Certified Personal Trainer® (CPT®), Tactical Strength and Conditioning Facilitator® (TSAC-F®), and Certified Special Populations Specialist® (CSPS®). The organization produced decades of peer-reviewed research journals and magazines aimed at providing fitness professionals with evidence-based strength and conditioning guidelines. NSCA® certifications are highly recognized in the fitness industry and generally very well respected. The main goal of the NSCA® is to supply the health and fitness world with the best research-based information on fitness and sports performance for the benefit of all fitness professionals.

NSCA®–CSCS® Test Details

The NSCA®—CSCS® exam is a computer-based, multiple-choice exam separated into two sections, each of which is further split into domains. The two sections include a scientific foundations section and a practical application section. Both sections include an additional fifteen questions that are unscored and regarded as potential examination questions for the future. These are not indicated on the test and are mixed in with the rest of the scored questions, so you must answer all the questions on the exam.

What's on the NSCA®–CSCS®?

Section 1: Scientific Foundations

Domain	Number of Questions	Percentage of Test
Exercise Science	59	74%
Nutrition	21	26%
Total:	95 total questions (including 15 unscored)	1 hour and 30 minutes

Section 2: Practical/Applied

Domain	Number of Questions	Percentage of Test
Exercise Technique	38	35%
Program Design	39	35%
Organization and Administration	13	12%
Testing and Evaluation	20	18%
Total:	125 total questions (including 15 unscored)	2 hours and 30 minutes

The first section, Scientific Foundations, covers exercise science and nutrition. Candidates will be tested on anatomy, exercise physiology as it relates to the major body systems, biomechanics, nutrition, hydration, and weight management, among other topics. Candidates have one and a half hours to complete this portion of the CSCS® exam.

The second section, Practical/Applied, is split into four domains and includes various videos and pictures relating to different exercise techniques, exercise testing, and functional anatomy. Review your knowledge of performing and interpreting the results of subjective assessments, physical assessments, and body composition assessments. Expect questions on training methods; periodization; the principles of specificity, overload, and variation; program design for special populations; and other issues. There may also be questions about proper cueing techniques, safe training and spotting practices, and signs of contraindications. Like Section 1, this section contains fifteen unscored questions. They are interspersed throughout the exam and are not indicated, so you must answer every question. Candidates are afforded two and a half hours to complete this portion of the exam.

To take the exam, a candidate must have a bachelor's degree or be currently enrolled as a college senior at an accredited institution. He or she must also have certification in CPR and AED. The exam is administered by Pearson VUE and offered at testing centers throughout the nation. Candidates should see the NSCA® for the most up-to-date information on fees and to register. There is a discount for NSCA® members. On test day, candidates must bring a valid photo ID and registration information.

ONE: Practice Test One

SCIENTIFIC FOUNDATIONS

READ THE QUESTION AND THEN CHOOSE THE MOST CORRECT ANSWER.

1. Which vitamins act as hormones that bind to cellular receptors and regulate cellular processes?

   A) vitamins A and D

   B) vitamins D and K

   C) vitamins C and E

   D) folate and B-12

2. Bones, ligaments, and cartilage are types of

   A) organs.

   B) connective tissues.

   C) cells.

   D) joints.

3. Where are posterior parts of the body positioned?

   A) on the front

   B) on the back

   C) on the top

   D) on the sides

4. The pulmonary vein carries

   A) deoxygenated blood from the body to the heart.

   B) air from the lungs to the blood.

   C) oxygenated blood from the lungs to the heart.

   D) deoxygenated blood from the heart to the lungs.

5. Ligaments adhere

   A) bone to bone.

   B) bone to muscle.

   C) muscle to muscle.

   D) cartilage to bone.

6. The pericardium is the

   A) innermost layer of the heart.

   B) middle layer of the heart.

   C) heart muscle.

   D) outermost layer of the heart.

7. The radius and ulna are bones found in which body part?

  A) the hand

  B) the forearm

  C) the leg

  D) the neck

8. Which joint allows for the most freedom of movement?

  A) ball-and-socket

  B) hinge

  C) saddle

  D) uniaxial

9. How many vertebrae does the spine have, excluding the coccygeal bones?

  A) 22

  B) 35

  C) 29

  D) 20

10. What does kyphosis of the spine mean?

  A) excessive anterior curvature

  B) excessive posterior curvature

  C) excessive lateral curvature

  D) excessive medial curvature

11. Lordosis is most commonly seen in which part of the spine?

  A) thoracic vertebrae

  B) sacral vertebrae

  C) coccygeal vertebrae

  D) lumbar vertebrae

12. Which of these is contained in the H-zone?

  A) myosin only

  B) actin only

  C) actin and myosin

  D) the Z-bands

13. Which exercise can improve bone mineral density?

  A) non-impact exercise

  B) swimming

  C) axial loading of the skeleton through weightlifting

  D) walking outside

14. What are the two contractile proteins found in sarcomeres?

  A) actin and myofibrils

  B) actin and motor units

  C) actin and myosin

  D) myosin and action potentials

15. What is the name of a single neuron and its associated skeletal muscle fibers that are innervated by that neuron?

  A) a muscle fiber

  B) the neuromuscular junction

  C) a sarcomere

  D) a motor unit

16. What are the three conditions that define the female athlete triad?

  A) bulimia nervosa, anemia, fatigue

  B) anorexia nervosa, anemia, dehydration

  C) disordered eating, amenorrhea, osteoporosis

  D) disordered eating, amenorrhea, anemia

17. Which of the following is represented by the volume of oxygen consumed during a particular activity measured in mL/kg body weight/minute?

  A) VO2 max

  B) exercise intensity

  C) VO2

  D) respiration rate

18. To maximize performance, a pre-exercise meal should be

   A) avoided, as it will weigh down the athlete.

   B) eaten just before competition to maximize available fuel.

   C) eaten one to six hours before competition.

   D) liquid in nature.

19. What is muscle hypertrophy?

   A) abnormally large muscle cells

   B) an increase in muscle cross section leading to increased strength

   C) excessively long muscle cells caused by anabolic steroids

   D) excessive muscle contractions leading to cramping

20. Anabolic steroids are illegal in competition and carry undesirable side effects and health risks. Which natural hormone do they mimic?

   A) testosterone

   B) estrogen

   C) aldosterone

   D) human growth hormone

21. What should older adults spend more time doing than younger adults in an exercise program?

   A) strength training

   B) power training

   C) high impact exercise

   D) warming up

22. What are the major mineral(s) in bone?

   A) calcium and zinc

   B) calcium, phosphate, and manganese

   C) calcium

   D) calcium, phosphate, and magnesium

23. Which best describes the process in the muscles during which the proteins actin and myosin form a connection to pull the thin actin filaments over the myosin, causing a shortening of the sarcomeres and a concomitant shortening of the muscles, known as muscular contraction?

   A) sliding myofibril theory

   B) sliding filament theory

   C) sliding muscle theory

   D) sliding motor unit theory

24. Which of the following is NOT a form of blood doping, which is illegal?

   A) transfusions

   B) erythropoietin

   C) synthetic oxygen carriers

   D) iron supplements

25. Which drugs are sometimes used by athletes attempting to conceal illegal drug use?

   A) peptide hormones

   B) diuretics

   C) beta blockers

   D) TNF-a inhibitors

26. Which mineral is a component of the thyroid hormone?

   A) selenium

   B) iodine

   C) magnesium

   D) cobalt

27. Delayed onset muscle soreness (DOMS) is caused by

   A) lactic acid buildup in the muscles.

   B) static stretching.

   C) micro-tears in the muscle fibers.

   D) a sedentary lifestyle.

28. Saturated fat should constitute no more than 10 percent of daily caloric intake.

For a 2,000 kcal daily intake, what is the maximum number of grams of saturated fat that should be consumed?

A) 200 grams

B) 22 grams

C) 20 grams

D) 2 grams

29. High blood LDL cholesterol is detrimental to cardiovascular health; soluble fiber can lower LDL cholesterol levels. Which of the following foods contain soluble fiber?

A) oatmeal, fruits, and beans

B) meat and dairy products

C) whole wheat, brown rice, and seeds

D) vegetable oils

30. Waist circumference is a measure of abdominal obesity. Measurements greater than which of the following are considered unhealthy for men and for women?

A) 40 inches for men and 35 inches for women

B) 40 inches for both men and women

C) 45 inches for men and 40 inches for women

D) 45 inches for both men and women

31. Which of these is a proprioceptor found within the musculotendinous junction that senses the amount of force being placed on the muscle and functions to prevent excessive forceful contractions of the muscle via autogenic inhibition?

A) Golgi tendon organs

B) muscle spindle fibers

C) motor units

D) action potentials

32. Ventral and anterior are similar terms because they both imply something positioned

A) toward the back of the body.

B) toward the front of the body.

C) toward the sides of the body.

D) toward the feet.

33. Which athlete will benefit from fast-twitch muscle fibers the most?

A) marathoners

B) 1500-meter swimmers

C) Olympic sprinters

D) cross-country cyclists

34. What do slow-twitch muscle fibers contain more of than fast-twitch muscle fibers?

A) mitochondria

B) anaerobic capacity

C) force production capability

D) types of fibers

35. Which two actions do the quadriceps muscles perform?

A) knee flexion and hip flexion

B) knee extension and hip flexion

C) knee flexion and hip extension

D) knee extension and hip extension

36. A phase during the neuromuscular stimulation process that involves myosin crossbridges attaching and pulling actin filaments closer together, resulting in a shortening of the sarcomeres and subsequent muscle fibers, refers to which phase of muscle contraction?

A) the relaxation phase

B) the contraction phase

C) the recharge phase

D) the eccentric phase

37. The triceps perform elbow extension in which plane?

A) frontal

B) transverse

C) sagittal

D) oblique

38. What is the action of the gastrocnemius muscle?

A) ankle dorsiflexion

B) ankle extension

C) ankle plantar flexion

D) ankle flexion

39. Which of the answer choices refers to a muscular contraction in which the resistance and force are even and no movement is taking place?

A) concentric muscle contraction

B) isotonic muscle contraction

C) isokinetic muscle contraction

D) isometric muscle contraction

40. Which term describes when a joint is decreasing its angle by muscular contraction?

A) extension

B) circumduction

C) flexion

D) rotation

41. An example of a muscular stabilizer during an exercise is

A) the latissimus dorsi during a lat pulldown exercise.

B) the gluteus medius during the box step-up exercise.

C) the biceps brachii during the biceps curl exercise.

D) the quadriceps during a squat exercise.

42. Collections of tissues throughout the body with a similar function are referred to as

A) tissues.

B) posterior.

C) organ systems.

D) organs.

43. Which of the following refers to the optimal muscular length at the level of the sarcomere for maximum force potential of the muscle?

A) length-tension relationship

B) force-couple relationship

C) sliding filament theory

D) motor unit recruitment

44. What is muscular hypertrophy?

A) an increase in the number of muscle cells

B) an increase in the size of the muscle cells

C) a decrease in the size of the muscle cells

D) an increase in the length of the muscle cells

45. Which of the following feeds the right atrium with deoxygenated blood from the body?

A) the superior and inferior vena cava

B) the carotid artery

C) the aorta

D) the lungs

46. Because of an increased Q-angle, female athletes are at a higher risk of medial knee injuries in which sport(s)?

A) rock climbing

B) basketball and volleyball

C) ice hockey

D) snowboarding

47. Distal means
    A) toward the axial skeleton.
    B) toward the skull.
    C) away from the axial skeleton.
    D) toward the midline of the body.

48. The trachea carries air to the
    A) bronchi.
    B) mouth.
    C) bronchioles.
    D) alveoli.

49. Which of the following is found in blood and aids in clotting?
    A) red blood cells
    B) platelets
    C) white blood cells
    D) water

50. Which of the following is a muscle that helps to create a pressure differential in the abdomen and chest, allowing air to flow into and out of the lungs when contracting and relaxing, respectively?
    A) abdominals
    B) pectoralis major
    C) pectoralis minor
    D) diaphragm

51. Where does digestion begin?
    A) stomach
    B) esophagus
    C) mouth
    D) small intestine

52. The central nervous system is made up of
    A) the brain and nerves.
    B) the brain and spinal cord.
    C) the brain and proprioceptors.
    D) the spinal cord and nerves.

53. What muscular action occurs as a limb is pulled toward the midline of the body?
    A) abduction
    B) extension
    C) pronation
    D) adduction

54. What is multiple sclerosis?
    A) a disease associated with memory loss and dementia that occurs later in life
    B) a disease affecting bone mineral density
    C) a disease that affects the myelin sheaths that surround axons on a neuron
    D) a disease that damages the nucleus of neurons

55. When the nervous system sends an impulse for muscular twitch and then immediately sends another before the muscle has time to relax, it is referred to as
    A) motor unit recruitment.
    B) neuromuscular adaptation.
    C) summation.
    D) a stimulus.

56. What are disordered heart rhythms called?
    A) arrhythmias
    B) amenorrhea
    C) hypertension
    D) atherosclerosis

57. What are the two important types of hormones associated with exercise?
    A) anabolic and testosterone
    B) anabolic and IGF
    C) anabolic and epinephrine
    D) anabolic and catabolic

58. Which of the following is an organ associated with controlling the release of chemical substances, known as hormones, for the regulation of metabolic processes, growth, development, sexual reproduction, and other bodily functions?

A) a hormone

B) the brain

C) testosterone

D) a gland

59. The hypothalamus controls

A) autonomic nervous system function and the connection between the central nervous system and endocrine system.

B) the peripheral nervous system and associated nerves.

C) the musculoskeletal system and voluntary skeletal muscle.

D) human growth and development.

60. Which of the following is the part of the uterus that passes nutrition and nourishment to the fetus from the mother via the umbilicus during pregnancy?

A) ovaries

B) placenta

C) testis

D) pineal gland

61. A force-time curve for an isometric exercise will likely

A) not indicate any increase on the axis of the force.

B) spike dramatically and then return to normal levels within a short time period.

C) increase and then stable out due to the exercise being held for time at a specific force.

D) have a short spike in force, a drop, and then a stabilization.

62. The BMI might NOT be an accurate indicator of a healthy weight

A) when the individual is tall.

B) when the individual is short.

C) if the individual is a strength trainer.

D) if the individual is sedentary.

63. The components of a lever system include

A) the force, the resistance, and the weight.

B) the muscles, the resistance, and the force.

C) the fulcrum, the resistance, and the weight.

D) the fulcrum, the resistance, and the force.

64. What is the most common type of lever system the human body uses?

A) a first-class lever

B) The body does not use levers.

C) a second-class lever

D) a third-class lever

65. Which of the following best describes Newton's second law of motion?

A) force = mass × power

B) force = mass × acceleration

C) Momentum and impulse are the same.

D) Power and work are the same.

66. What is the amount of muscular force (force) needed to move an object through a joint's angular range of motion (distance)?

A) rotational power

B) angular velocity

C) rotational work

D) momentum

67. Which of the following best describes the maximal rate at which lactic acid due to exercise can be buffered from the blood stream?

A) the lactate threshold

B) the Krebs cycle

C) the phosphagen system

D) the anaerobic energy system

68. Approximately how much caloric expenditure through exercise is recommended to lose about one pound per week?

A) 500 kcal/week

B) 1,000 kcal/week

C) 1,500 kcal/week

D) 2,000 kcal/week

69. How might a rock climber and figure skater vary in muscle mass?

A) They should have similar distributions of muscle mass.

B) The rock climber will have stronger abdominal muscles.

C) The figure skater will likely have more lower body muscle mass.

D) The figure skater will likely have more upper body muscle mass.

70. What are the dietary protein recommendations for sedentary individuals, those engaging in endurance exercise, and strength trainers?

A) The RDA for protein intake is 0.8 g/kg body weight.

B) 0.8 g/kg, 1.6 g/kg, and 2.2 g/kg, respectively

C) 1.2 g/kg

D) 0.8 – 0.9 g/kg, 1.2 – 1.4 g/kg, and 1.6 – 1.7 g/kg, respectively

71. How does lean body mass differ from fat-free mass?

A) Lean body mass includes just muscle.

B) Lean body mass does not include water.

C) Fat-free mass includes the brain.

D) Lean body mass includes some fatty organs/tissues—like the brain and spinal cord—while fat-free mass does not.

72. What are the three components of the female athlete triad?

A) amenorrhea, muscle growth, and reduced bone mineral density

B) amenorrhea, reduced bone mineral density, and fatigue

C) fatigue, reduced bone mineral density, and disordered eating habits

D) amenorrhea, reduced bone mineral density, and disordered eating habits

73. IGF-1 helps promote

A) muscle maintenance and repair.

B) muscle energy stores.

C) peak strength output.

D) the rate of muscular contraction.

74. Which is **not** a type of cartilage?

A) hyaline

B) fibrocartilage

C) elastic

D) ligaments

75. Which population has difficulty regulating body temperature?

A) children

B) women

C) older adults

D) men

76. Disordered eating in female athletes can lead to

A) reduced bone mineral density and loss of menstrual cycle.

B) improved health.

C) muscle mass development.

D) improved fitness performance.

77. The musculoskeletal system is comprised of levers to

A) digest food.

B) create red blood cells.

C) create movement.

D) conduct nervous impulses.

78. How does age influence the heart?

A) It increases cardiac output.

B) It increases blood pressure.

C) It decreases maximum heart rate.

D) It decreases resting heart rate.

79. How many different amino acids are involved in protein metabolism?

A) twenty

B) ten

C) eight

D) twenty-one

80. What is the difference between a macromineral and a micromineral?

A) Macrominerals are larger than microminerals.

B) Macrominerals are required in the diet in larger quantities than microminerals.

C) Macrominerals bind together to form large complexes.

D) Microminerals are derived from microbial organisms in the gut.

81. Which vitamin or vitamin precursor is NOT an antioxidant?

A) vitamin E

B) vitamin C

C) beta-carotene

D) vitamin K

82. Which is an example of a convergent muscle?

A) biceps brachii

B) extensor digitorum longus

C) rectus abdominis

D) pectoralis major

83. Deficiencies of which vitamins or minerals can cause megaloblastic anemia?

A) thiamine

B) folate and vitamin B-12

C) iron

D) copper

84. Which type of athletes are at risk for iron-deficiency anemia?

A) both strength and endurance athletes

B) male athletes

C) strength athletes, female athletes, and vegetarians

D) endurance athletes, female athletes, and vegetarians

85. Which of the following is true? Vibrating belts and electric stimulators

A) burn calories with little effort.

B) can be used to lose fat in specific body areas.

C) are a useful addition to exercise.

D) do not burn significant calories and are not capable of eliminating fat in specific body areas.

86. Which macronutrients are the major fuels for exercise?

   A) carbohydrates and fats

   B) protein and carbohydrates

   C) protein and fats

   D) carbohydrates, fats, and protein

87. What is glycemic index?

   A) a measure of the energy density of a food

   B) a measure of the rate of glycogen depletion during exercise

   C) a measure of the rise in blood glucose caused by a standard amount of a food

   D) a measure of the percentage of kcal from carbohydrates in a food

88. Which electrolytes are responsible for the transmission of electrical signals across nerve and muscle cell membranes?

   A) sodium and chloride

   B) potassium and chloride

   C) sodium and potassium

   D) sodium and magnesium

89. Which of the following refers to the larger heart chambers?

   A) atria

   B) ventricles

   C) veins

   D) valves

90. What does EPOC stand for?

   A) Excess Post-exercise Oxygen Creation

   B) Excess Post-exercise Oxygen Consumption

   C) Extreme Post-exercise Oxygen Consumption

   D) Excess Pre-exercise Oxygen Consumption

91. During exercise that lasts over one hour, how much fluid intake is recommended to maintain hydration?

   A) 20 – 36 oz. per hour

   B) 8 – 12 oz. per hour

   C) 10 – 15 oz. per hour

   D) 40 – 45 oz. per hour

92. Body composition in relation to a healthy weight

   A) is a measure of the relative proportions of carbohydrates, proteins, fat, and water in the body.

   B) is the percentage of fat-free mass versus fat mass in the body.

   C) is the percentage of bone versus soft tissue in the body.

   D) is the percentage of dry mass versus water in the body.

93. What is the function of saliva?

   A) hydration

   B) assist in the breakdown of food in the mouth

   C) nutrient absorption

   D) water absorption into the gut

94. The myelin sheath on axons helps

   A) speed up nervous transmission of electrical impulses.

   B) pass information to the dendrites.

   C) protect the nerve from damage caused by multiple sclerosis.

   D) prevent the onset of Alzheimer's disease.

95. Which of the following does NOT make weight loss more difficult?

   A) sleep deprivation

   B) type 2 diabetes

   C) certain antidepressants

   D) the drug metformin

PRACTICAL/APPLIED

Read the question and then choose the most correct answer.

1. Which test is the most effective for assessing speed, agility, and quickness?

   A) Rockport walk test

   B) push-up test

   C) hexagon test

   D) twelve-minute run test

2. What are the regions that are measured during the three-site skinfold assessment with a female client?

   A) chest, biceps, thigh

   B) triceps, suprailium, thigh

   C) subscapular, thigh, suprailium

   D) biceps, thigh, suprailium

3. All of the following tests are used to measure speed, agility, and quickness EXCEPT

   A) the 300-yard shuttle test.

   B) the LEFT

   C) the pro-agility test.

   D) the *t*-test.

4. Based on the principle of specificity, the fact that football players run one hundred yards at most should tell the trainer not to implement

   A) short-distance sprint intervals in the training program.

   B) long-distance running into the training program.

   C) power exercises for improved speed in the training program.

   D) muscular endurance exercises into the training program.

5. Which cycle is the shortest of a periodization program?

   A) the mesocycle

   B) the macrocycle

   C) the microcycle

   D) the preparatory period

6. Which of the following is generally NOT part of a fitness assessment?

   A) flexibility assessment

   B) static posture assessment

   C) daily caloric intake assessment

   D) cardiorespiratory capacity assessment

7. Movement assessments are used to test

   A) maximal force.

   B) core strength.

   C) agility and speed.

   D) dynamic posture.

8. Why is it important that fitness professionals obtain certification through a leading organization in the fitness industry?

   A) Trainers who are certified can make more money.

   B) Clients will often research the fitness professional's expertise and certifications.

   C) Trainers can guarantee client results with their certification.

   D) Certification is proof of the trainer's education.

9. A static stretch is held for how many seconds?

    A) 20 seconds

    B) 60 seconds

    C) 30 seconds

    D) 10 seconds

10. The body's response mechanism to absorbing too much physical stress in too short a time is called

    A) hypertension.

    B) hyperventilation.

    C) delayed onset muscle soreness.

    D) overtraining.

11. What are the legal parameters in which all credentialed or licensed health professionals should work?

    A) scope of product

    B) legality of specialization

    C) scope of practice

    D) terms of work

12. A network of licensed, certified, or registered professionals who provide healthcare resources to the general population is called what?

    A) allied healthcare continuum

    B) training continuum

    C) health professionals

    D) health maintenance professionals

13. Which assessment would be most appropriate for a sixty-five-year-old client who wants to lower his or her blood pressure?

    A) bench press test

    B) hexagon test

    C) Rockport walk test

    D) three-hundred-yard shuttle test

14. If a client complains of experiencing pain or injury during a session, a trainer should refer the client to

    A) the client's physician.

    B) a friend.

    C) a massage therapist.

    D) no one.

15. During the BESS, which of the following actions does NOT result in error points being given?

    A) opening of the eyes

    B) remaining in the proper position for twenty seconds

    C) moving hands off of the hips

    D) lifting the ball or heel of the foot off of the testing surface

16. Which type of exercises typically activates smaller muscle groups and is used for rehabilitative purposes?

    A) core exercises

    B) open kinetic chain exercises

    C) PNF stretching

    D) assistance exercises

17. A lifestyle questionnaire should NOT include questions which pertain to which of the following?

    A) sleep

    B) stress

    C) friends

    D) smoking

18. Clients with arthritis may have decreased

    A) joint pain.

    B) motivation to exercise.

    C) joint range of motion.

    D) muscular atrophy.

19. The allied healthcare continuum (AHC) includes all the following professionals, EXCEPT

A) a nurse.

B) a psychologist.

C) an occupational therapist.

D) a psychic.

20. Which of the following is NOT a muscular strength, endurance, and power assessment?

A) long jump test

B) Margaria-Kalamen test

C) star excursion test

D) reactive strength index

21. A professional trainer would wear which of following?

A) khaki pants or jeans

B) tasteful athletic attire

C) revealing athletic attire

D) strong cologne or perfume

22. Which tool is used to manually assess blood pressure?

A) handheld bioelectrical impedance device

B) sphygmomanometer

C) calipers

D) scale

23. How should the trainer modify abdominal exercises, such as the crunch, for pregnant clients?

A) No modification is necessary.

B) Reduce the range of motion dramatically.

C) Pregnant clients are not allowed to perform abdominal exercises.

D) Have the client seated slightly upright.

24. The second transition period is a period of

A) high-intensity training.

B) sports-specific training.

C) no physical activity at all.

D) active recovery involving non-specific recreational activity.

25. Which test helps determine an individual's ability to change direction and stabilize the body at high speeds?

A) hexagon test

B) t-test

C) pro-agility test

D) vertical jump test

26. Core exercises are classified into two subcategories: structural and _____.

A) open

B) assistance

C) power

D) static

27. Performing _____ stretching in a circuit can be a cardio warm-up.

A) static

B) passive

C) dynamic

D) active

28. If a client has a muscle imbalance, what should she be directed to do in her warm-up?

A) active stretching before static stretching

B) SMR or foam roll before dynamic stretching

C) static stretching before cardio warm-up

D) SMR or foam roll before static stretching

29. A superset in a training program refers to

   A) performing an exercise and gradually increasing load, then decreasing load per set.

   B) performing multiple sets of a single exercise with intermittent rest periods.

   C) performing an exercise and then immediately performing another exercise utilizing the antagonist or opposite muscle groups.

   D) performing a series of different exercises in a row with a rest period at the end of the series.

30. High-volume and low-load muscular endurance training can cause fatigue and should be saved for the

   A) in-season.

   B) off-season.

   C) competitive period.

   D) second transition period.

31. Performing a specific number of repetitions through the full range of motion is called

   A) a workout.

   B) the load.

   C) overload.

   D) a set.

32. The last part of a warm-up should consist of what type of stretching?

   A) static stretching

   B) PNF stretching

   C) dynamic stretching

   D) SMR stretching

33. What is a regression for a push press?

   A) seated dumbbell shoulder press

   B) standing upright row

   C) low pulley row

   D) push-up

34. How many spotters are needed for a dumbbell shoulder press?

   A) none

   B) 2

   C) 3

   D) 1

35. What method can assist the fitness professional in determining if a client is potentially overtraining?

   A) ask the client if he thinks he is overtraining

   B) ask one of the client's relatives for an opinion on whether the client is overtraining

   C) keep detailed records of the client's training outcomes and responses to training

   D) send the client to another fitness professional

36. Which of the following refers to the degree to which a test or test item measures what is supposed to be measured?

   A) relativity

   B) honesty

   C) validity

   D) strength

37. A dynamic warm-up for a field hockey player should include these three things:

A) static stretching, dynamic stretching, and cardiovascular exercise

B) dynamic stretching, single-muscle group exercises, and plyometrics

C) five minutes of aerobic exercise, dynamic stretching, and specific movement patterns of the workout

D) dynamic stretching, PNF stretching, and foam rolling

38. What is the primary sensor in autogenic inhibition?

A) muscle spindles

B) Golgi tendon organ

C) tendon

D) ligaments

39. Loads of 90 percent of 1RM require a rest period of how long for proper recovery?

A) thirty seconds or less

B) ninety seconds or less

C) one minute

D) three minutes or more

40. A foam roller is used for what type of training?

A) PNF stretching

B) active stretching

C) power training

D) self-myofascial release

41. Which of the following is NOT a positive body language indicator?

A) nodding slowly or quickly

B) leaning forward

C) wringing hands

D) firm handshake

42. Resistance training programs for children and adolescents should focus on

A) increasing weight lifted.

B) specific and repetitive movements.

C) high-intensity exercise.

D) proper technique and form.

43. Which exercise may require a spotter?

A) barbell deadlift

B) medicine ball slam

C) back-loaded squat

D) walking lunges

44. When meeting with a client, the trainer should exude

A) cockiness, enthusiasm, and joy.

B) confidence, enthusiasm, and professionalism.

C) confidence, assertiveness, and likeability.

D) pride, love, and goodness.

45. Which of the following assessments does NOT measure body fat percentage?

A) dual-energy x-ray absorptiometry (DEXA)

B) body mass index (BMI)

C) near-infrared interactance

D) air displacement plethysmography (BOD POD)

46. A grip used primarily in parallel bar or dumbbell pushing and pulling movements where the thumbs stay up and the palms face each other is:

A) supinated grip

B) alternating grip

C) false grip

D) neutral grip

47. To ensure accuracy of the results, the resting heart rate should be taken at what time of the day?

   A) before a workout

   B) at the end of the work day

   C) upon rising in the morning

   D) while resting during a workout

48. Which grip is overhanded?

   A) alternated grip

   B) supinated grip

   C) pronated grip

   D) clean grip

49. When clients who are new to running start a running program, they may benefit from a jogging and walking work-to-rest ratio of what?

   A) 1:5

   B) 2:1

   C) 3:1

   D) 1:1

50. What joint motion would be used in the frontal plane of motion?

   A) abduction/adduction

   B) flexion/extension

   C) rotational

   D) vertical

51. A tuck jump is an example of what type of training?

   A) plyometrics training

   B) explosive training

   C) resistance training

   D) kettlebell training

52. In a standing or sitting position, a client should maintain which three points of contact?

   A) shoulders, calves, heels

   B) head, shoulders, glutes

   C) head, glutes, calves

   D) shoulders, glutes, heels

53. What type of aerobic exercise should be included in programs focused on general health benefits?

   A) running only

   B) cycling and swimming only

   C) all modes are beneficial

   D) general health benefits do not require aerobic exercise

54. The gastrocnemius is another name for what muscle?

   A) forearm

   B) thigh

   C) calf

   D) neck

55. Personal attributes, which can hinder exercise adherence, include all of the following, EXCEPT what?

   A) age

   B) accessibility

   C) time

   D) fitness level

56. A circuit-training program involving a careful selection of varying muscle groups to minimize rest periods is called

   A) horizontal loading.

   B) single set.

   C) interval training.

   D) vertical loading.

57. _____ is the body's ability to react to a cue that propels a change in direction.

A) Agility
B) Quickness
C) Readiness
D) Stabilization

58. Strength training should follow a progressive plan with three tiers, which are _____, _____, and _____.

A) power, muscle, matter
B) strength, power, hard
C) stabilization, strength, power
D) stabilization, body, strength

59. Which of the following is NOT true of the drawing-in maneuver?

A) It aids in core activation.
B) It maintains neutral posturing.
C) It is used for all core exercises.
D) It stretches the hip flexors.

60. Why might plyometrics not be advisable for individuals who are overweight or obese?

A) They develop muscular power.
B) They are not fun.
C) They are too easy.
D) They place excessive force on the joints.

61. How many points of contact should a client have when lying in a semi-supine position?

A) 7
B) 3
C) 4
D) 5

62. When exercising for weight loss, the mode of cardiovascular exercise

A) is not important.
B) should be specific.
C) should be steady state.
D) must be low impact.

63. Plyometrics training primarily focuses on explosive movement and full range of motion, while speed, agility, and quickness training keeps the exercises _____.

A) compact
B) slow
C) painful
D) controlled

64. A barbell deadlift or a rear loaded squat can be considered _____ exercises.

A) structural
B) power
C) agility
D) assistance

65. Which assessment is used to assess weight relative to height?

A) waist-to-hip ratio
B) air displacement plethysmography (BOD POD)
C) body mass index
D) skinfold measurements

66. What type of training uses controlled instability to increase proprioception?

A) plyometrics
B) cardio training
C) free weight training
D) core training

67. Ice skaters are used for what type of training?

   A) plyometrics

   B) stabilization

   C) free weight

   D) stretching

68. The 1RM test measures the client's

   A) ability to perform an exercise at the maximal effort of strength for a single repetition.

   B) weight utilized for all exercises in the program.

   C) target heart rate zone.

   D) ability to perform an exercise at submaximal efforts for multiple repetitions.

69. Treadmills, elliptical trainers, and rowing machines are used for what type of training?

   A) functional training

   B) resistance training

   C) power training

   D) aerobic training

70. A push jerk is what type of core exercise?

   A) structural exercise

   B) stability exercise

   C) power exercise

   D) standing exercise

71. Detraining occurs more rapidly

   A) in cardiovascular health.

   B) in muscular strength.

   C) in clients who have previously trained.

   D) in professional athletes.

72. Which of the following assessments are used as indicators of a client's general fitness and overall health?

   A) cardiorespiratory assessments

   B) movement assessments

   C) muscular endurance assessments

   D) physiological assessments

73. Which of the following is most likely to cause a muscular imbalance of the upper body?

   A) a training program that utilizes alternating push-and-pull exercises

   B) a bodyweight training program that includes exercises for the chest, back, core, and legs

   C) a well-balanced yoga routine with a trained instructor

   D) a unilateral training program emphasizing strengthening of the pectorals and anterior deltoids

74. A false grip is

   A) an underhanded grip.

   B) where the thumb is wrapped around the bar along with the fingers.

   C) where the thumb is wrapped around the bar on the opposite side of the fingers.

   D) where the thumb is facing the ceiling and the palms are toward the body.

75. When should static stretching be performed in a workout?

   A) prior to exercise

   B) before the plyometrics

   C) before the cardiovascular exercise

   D) at the end of the workout

76. A typical mesocycle may last
    A) six to twelve weeks.
    B) one week.
    C) an entire year.
    D) nearly two years.

77. A floor crunch is a regression for what core exercise?
    A) reverse crunch
    B) plank hold
    C) hip bridge
    D) ball crunch

78. Which of the following is NOT an example of relapse prevention and recovery plans?
    A) use the ABC model of behavior to identify triggers
    B) plan a weekly menu and shopping list to eliminate the need for a fast food meal
    C) do NOT focus on fault
    D) create a contingency plan for social outings

79. Which connect chain checkpoint compensation reveals lower crossed syndrome?
    A) shoulders
    B) foot and ankle
    C) head and cervical spine
    D) lumbo/pelvic/hip complex

80. The Karvonen formula is used to calculate
    A) maximum heart rate.
    B) target heart rate.
    C) resting heart rate.
    D) heart rate recovery.

81. Why should power exercises be performed prior to muscular endurance exercises?
    A) to promote flexibility
    B) power exercises are lower intensity and should be performed first
    C) muscular endurance exercises are higher intensity and should be performed last
    D) power exercises require high levels of technique, and muscular endurance exercises can cause fatigue and decreased performance quality

82. How might a goaltender's training program differ from that of any other position in soccer?
    A) The specific movements will involve more forward movement speed development.
    B) The goaltender will perform more steady-state cardiovascular exercise.
    C) The goaltender will perform more exercises to develop kicking and core power.
    D) The specific movements will involve more lateral movement speed development.

83. Developing a training program to achieve a specific goal determined by the trainer and client refers to what?
    A) progression
    B) regression
    C) detraining
    D) specificity

84. Free weight benches with barbells should accommodate

   A) at least two spotters.

   B) at least three spotters.

   C) at least one spotter.

   D) at least the person lifting the barbell.

85. Which answer describes why the following is NOT a SMART goal?

   The client wants to lose twenty-five pounds in two months.

   A) The goal is not specific.

   B) The goal is not time-stamped.

   C) The goal is not realistic.

   D) The goal is not measurable.

86. What is an appropriate amount to increase cardiovascular training variables?

   A) 0.5 percent

   B) 10 percent

   C) 11 percent

   D) 15 percent

87. Once the body has detrained cardiovascularly in a trained individual, how long does it take to recover to the same fitness level?

   A) It can take several months.

   B) It takes only a few days.

   C) Cardiovascular detraining does not happen.

   D) It takes several years.

88. During a gait assessment, the personal trainer should use the lateral view to check which kinetic chain checkpoint?

   A) lumbo/pelvic/hip complex

   B) head, low back, and shoulders

   C) knees

   D) ankles/feet

89. A macrocycle includes

   A) only the in-season program.

   B) the entirety of a training periodization.

   C) only off-season training.

   D) only the preparatory period of training.

90. Detraining occurs more quickly in

   A) resistance training gains.

   B) cardiovascular training gains.

   C) men.

   D) women.

91. Excessive training frequency can cause

   A) rapid gains in fitness.

   B) stress reduction.

   C) increased training intensity.

   D) overuse injuries.

92. What type of aerobic endurance training is the 10-kilometer row?

   A) interval

   B) zone training

   C) anaerobic endurance

   D) steady state

93. What is the primary mover for a wrist curl?

   A) triceps

   B) forearm

   C) shoulder

   D) biceps

94. Which of the following is NOT an example of the self-monitoring behavior modification technique?

   A) diet journaling

   B) activity tracking

   C) rewarding completion of a goal

   D) incorporating weekly weigh-ins

95. With resistance training, the intensity increases as the

    A) weight decreases.

    B) volume increases.

    C) weight increases.

    D) repetitions increase.

96. How might the trainer progress an already difficult exercise, such as a single-leg squat?

    A) There is no further progression.

    B) Add a box to sit down on.

    C) Add weight with a vest or dumbbells.

    D) Pick a new exercise to perform.

97. How long should the rest period be between sets of deadlifts at five repetitions and heavy loads?

    A) one minute

    B) less than thirty seconds

    C) three minutes

    D) six minutes

98. In which situation would a personal trainer need to immediately refer a client to a medical professional?

    A) a client complains of lower back pain

    B) a client complains of anterior knee pain

    C) a client has had recent complications with cardiac disease

    D) a client does not feel well

99. Which postural misalignment is characterized by rounded shoulders and a forward head position?

    A) lower crossed syndrome

    B) upper crossed syndrome

    C) pronation distortion

    D) knee valgus

100. Program design for weight management should include

    A) resistance training and nutrition.

    B) cardiovascular training and nutrition.

    C) nutrition only.

    D) warm-up, resistance training, cardiovascular training, nutrition, cooldown, and recovery methods.

101. To reduce the risk of liability in a potential lawsuit, fitness professionals should require that new clients complete which of the following?

    A) medical history forms, a liability waiver, informed consent to exercise, and a PAR-Q

    B) medical history forms, favorite hobbies, a bloodwork form, and a PAR-Q

    C) medical history forms, a liability waiver, informed consent, and a bloodwork form

    D) medical history forms, a liability waiver, a PAR-Q, and a fitness assessment

102. Which of the following is the strongest indicator of how a client's cardiorespiratory system is responding and adapting to exercise?

    A) resting heart rate

    B) 1.5-mile run

    C) body composition

    D) muscular strength test

103. Income is categorized as which type of barrier to exercise adherence?

    A) personal attribute

    B) environmental factor

    C) physical-activity factor

    D) core factor

104. Which compensations should the personal trainer look for at the foot and ankle while observing the client from the anterior view?

A) not adducted or abducted

B) not flattened or externally rotated

C) not anteriorly or posteriorly rotated

D) neither tilted nor rotated

105. Which test is most suitable to assess lower body strength?

A) long jump

B) barbell squat

C) overhead squat

D) hexagon

106. During the single-leg squat assessment, which of the following should NOT describe an individual's posture?

A) The foot should be pointed straight ahead.

B) The ankle, knee, and lumbo/pelvic/hip complex should remain in a neutral position.

C) The shoulders should round forward, and the neck should rest on the chest.

D) The knee should remain in line with the foot.

107. A personal trainer's attire should be

A) tasteful and modest fitness clothing.

B) jeans and a t-shirt.

C) tight and revealing.

D) sweaty and worn.

108. Verbal communication comprises only _____ of how we express ourselves.

A) 7 percent

B) 10 percent

C) 55 percent

D) 38 percent

109. What type of cardiovascular training is most specific to a golfer?

A) sprint training

B) a walking program with varying inclines

C) spin classes

D) long-distance steady-state jogging

110. Which of the following is NOT among the ways personal trainers can earn CECs?

A) college courses

B) industry specialization certification

C) blog contributions

D) structured learning modules from accredited programs

111. During clinical exercise testing protocols at a medical facility, it is the certified fitness professional's responsibility to

A) administer testing procedures under the guidance of a physician.

B) administer medical treatment and medical procedures to the client.

C) diagnose the client's symptoms based on the exercise test.

D) supervise the physician and staff during testing protocols.

112. Program design for clients with chronic back pain should emphasize

A) upper body resistance training.

B) core muscle endurance and flexibility training.

C) lower body resistance training.

D) avoiding the low back entirely.

113. Proper maintenance and routine checking of fitness equipment can help prevent

  A) client dissatisfaction.

  B) environmental emergencies.

  C) negligence lawsuits.

  D) overtraining injuries.

114. One major advantage of zone training in cardiovascular exercise programs is that

  A) it is always low intensity and safe.

  B) the mode does not change so it is easy to remember.

  C) it provides variety in cardiovascular training, which helps with program compliance.

  D) it takes less time than steady-state aerobic training.

115. Minimizing opportunities that trigger unwanted behavior in order to maximize desired behavior is called

  A) stimulus control.

  B) socio-ecological theory.

  C) self-monitoring.

  D) locus of control.

116. If a relapse occurs, using positive self-talk to acknowledge successes is an example of which behavioral change tool?

  A) cognitive coping

  B) social support

  C) relapse prevention

  D) time management

117. Which behavior change model focuses on understanding the relationship between a person and his or her environment?

  A) readiness-to-change model

  B) social cognitive theory model

  C) theory of planned behavior

  D) socio-ecological model

118. Which of the following is NOT a legal or ethical standard for personal trainers?

  A) denying culpability for personal actions

  B) maintaining accurate and honest notes for each client

  C) not discriminating based on race, gender, creed, age, ability, or sexual orientation

  D) complying with sexual harassment standards for both clients and peers

119. People who believe that life is controlled by things that happen to them have _____ locus of control.

  A) an internal

  B) an intrinsic

  C) an external

  D) a skewed

120. Low self-efficacy and external locus of control dominate people in the _____ phase; they believe their situations are hopeless and they would rather ignore them.

  A) preparation

  B) precontemplation

  C) action

  D) termination

121. In the relapse prevention and recovery plan techniques of behavior change, the ABC model of behavior helps to identify _____ for unwanted or desired activities.

   A) triggers

   B) obsessions

   C) irritants

   D) successes

122. Miscellaneous personal trainer's insurance covers which type of claims?

   A) defamation

   B) wrongful invasion of privacy

   C) wrongful termination

   D) bodily injury

123. Which term describes positive feedback emphasizing a specific aspect of an individual's behavior or task?

   A) kinesthetic feedback

   B) positive reinforcement

   C) targeted praise

   D) non-verbal communication

124. What percentage of 1RM should muscular power exercises be performed at?

   A) between 65 and 75%

   B) between 80 and 100%

   C) between 0 and 60%

   D) between 75 and 90%

125. Periods in a periodization follow this order:

   A) preparatory period, competitive period, first transition period, second transition period

   B) macrocycle, microcycle, mesocycle

   C) competitive period, first transition period, second transition period, preparatory period

   D) preparatory period, first transition period, competitive period, second transition period

PRACTICE TEST ONE SCIENTIFIC FOUNDATIONS ANSWER KEY

1. **A)** **Correct.** Vitamins A and D regulate a large variety of cellular processes as hormones.

    B) Incorrect. Vitamin K does not act as a hormone.

    C) Incorrect. Vitamins C and E are antioxidants, not hormones.

    D) Incorrect. Folate and B-12 are not hormones.

2. A) Incorrect. These are types of tissues, not organs.

    B) **Correct.** These are types of connective tissues.

    C) Incorrect. The terms listed in the question are known as tissues and are a collection of cells with a similar function.

    D) Incorrect. The three tissues listed in the question help make up the structure of joints, but they are only components.

3. A) Incorrect. This describes the position of anterior parts of the body.

    B) **Correct.** This is the correct position of posterior parts of the body.

    C) Incorrect. This describes the position of superior parts of the body.

    D) Incorrect. This is referring to the position of lateral parts of the body.

4. A) Incorrect. The pulmonary vein does not carry deoxygenated blood.

    B) Incorrect. The pulmonary vein does not oxygenate blood.

    C) **Correct.** The pulmonary vein carries oxygenated blood from the lungs to the heart.

    D) Incorrect. The pulmonary vein does not carry deoxygenated blood.

5. **A)** **Correct.** Ligaments adhere bone to bone.

    B) Incorrect. This refers to tendons.

    C) Incorrect. This is not the function of ligaments.

    D) Incorrect. This is not the function of ligaments.

6. A) Incorrect. This is the endocardium.

    B) Incorrect. This is the epicardium.

    C) Incorrect. This is myocardium.

    D) **Correct.** The pericardium is the outermost layer of the heart.

7. A) Incorrect. The carpals are the bones of the hand.

    B) **Correct.** The radius and ulna are the bones of the forearm.

    C) Incorrect. The femur, tibia, and fibula are found in the leg.

    D) Incorrect. The neck bones are the cervical vertebrae.

8. **A)** **Correct.** Ball-and-socket joints allow for the most freedom of movement.

    B) Incorrect. Hinge joints only allow for flexion and extension.

    C) Incorrect. Saddle joints do not allow rotation.

    D) Incorrect. Uniaxial joints only allow for movement through one plane of motion.

9. A) Incorrect. This is too few.

    B) Incorrect. This is too many.

    C) **Correct.** There are 29 vertebrae in the spine.

    D) Incorrect. This is too few.

10. A) Incorrect. This refers to lordosis.

    B) **Correct.** This is the definition of kyphosis.

    C) Incorrect. This refers to scoliosis.

    D) Incorrect. This does not refer to any of the discussed conditions.

11. A) Incorrect. Kyphosis is more common in the thoracic vertebrae.

    B) Incorrect. Lumbar is the most common area for lordosis.

C) Incorrect. This area is not common for lordosis.

D) **Correct.** The lumbar spine is the most common area for lordosis to occur.

12. A) **Correct.** The H-zone contains only thick myosin filaments.

B) Incorrect. The H-zone does not contain actin.

C) Incorrect. Actin is incorrect.

D) Incorrect. The H-zone does not contain Z-bands.

13. A) Incorrect. Non-impact exercise does not load the skeleton to elicit improvement to bone mineral density.

B) Incorrect. Swimming is a form of non-impact exercise.

C) **Correct.** Axial loading of the skeleton through weight lifting improves and maintains bone mineral density.

D) Incorrect. Though walking does involve impact, it is a relatively low-impact exercise.

14. A) Incorrect. Myofibrils is incorrect.

B) Incorrect. Motor units is incorrect.

C) **Correct.** Actin and myosin are contractile proteins in sarcomeres.

D) Incorrect. Action potentials is incorrect.

15. A) Incorrect. The muscle fiber is only a portion of this definition.

B) Incorrect. The neuromuscular junction is where the neuron and muscle fiber synapse.

C) Incorrect. This is a single unit of the muscle fiber.

D) **Correct.** This is the definition of a motor unit.

16. A) Incorrect. Although anemia is a risk for female athletes who do not eat much meat, it is not considered part of the female athlete triad, nor is fatigue part of the female   athlete triad.

B) Incorrect. Anemia and dehydration are not parts of the female athlete triad.

C) **Correct.** Female athletes in many sports feel pressured to stay extremely thin, which can lead to disordered eating and low energy intake. Nutrient deficiencies and extremely low body fat can lead to the loss of normal estrogen secretion, amenorrhea, and osteoporosis.

D) Incorrect. Anemia is not part of the female athlete triad.

17. A) Incorrect. This is the maximum rate of oxygen consumption an individual is capable of and improves with aerobic conditioning.

B) Incorrect. VO2 increases with a rise in exercise intensity.

C) **Correct.** VO2 is an abbreviation of the term volume of oxygen; it is defined as the volume of O2 consumed during any activity in mL/kg body weight/min.

D) Incorrect. Respiration rate is breaths/minute.

18. A) Incorrect. A pre-exercise meal is important to maximize glycogen storage and supply blood glucose.

B) Incorrect. This does not allow time for digestion and absorption of nutrients before the event.

C) **Correct.** This will allow for digestion, absorption of nutrients, and the incorporation of glucose into muscle and liver glycogen.

D) Incorrect. The meal does not need to be liquid in nature as there is time for digestion.

19. A) Incorrect. Hypertrophy is a normal increase in muscle size in response to exercise.

B) **Correct.** Muscle hypertrophy is the normal increase in muscle cross section leading to increased strength stimulated by exercise.

C) Incorrect. Hypertrophy is an increase in muscle cross section, not length.

D) Incorrect. Hypertrophy has nothing to do with cramping.

20.

A) **Correct.** Anabolic steroids are synthetic hormones that mimic the action of testosterone.

B) Incorrect. Estrogen is a steroid hormone, but anabolic steroids mimic testosterone.

C) Incorrect. Aldosterone is not involved in stimulating muscle growth.

D) Incorrect. Human growth hormone is a peptide hormone, not a steroid hormone.

21.

A) Incorrect. Spending more time strength training is safer in younger adults.

B) Incorrect. Due to the high intensity of the exercise, excessive amounts of power training can be dangerous to an older adult.

C) Incorrect. Some impact exercise is beneficial for older adults, but the higher the impact, the higher the risk of bone damage due to increased risk of osteoporosis with old age.

D) **Correct.** As people age, they should spend more time warming up before an exercise program.

22.

A) Incorrect. Zinc is present only in small quantities.

B) Incorrect. There is no significant amount of manganese in bone.

C) Incorrect. Calcium is not the only major mineral in bone.

D) **Correct.** Calcium and phosphate are most abundant, but magnesium is present in significant quantities also.

23.

A) Incorrect. Myofibril is incorrect.

B) **Correct.** This is the definition of the sliding filament theory.

C) Incorrect. Muscle is incorrect.

D) Incorrect. Motor unit is incorrect.

24.

A) Incorrect. Transfusing extra red blood cells is considered doping and is banned.

B) Incorrect. Erythropoietin (EPO) stimulates red blood cell production and is banned. EPO is also dangerous since it thickens the blood and may lead to stroke or heart attack.

C) Incorrect. Synthetic oxygen carriers could artificially increase the oxygen carrying capacity of the blood; they are banned.

D) **Correct.** Iron is a normal nutrient needed by the body and may require supplementation in anemic individuals. Supplementation is legal, and excess iron is generally excreted.

25.

A) Incorrect. Peptide hormones are used to enhance performance.

B) **Correct.** Diuretics increase urinary excretion and may be used to try to flush out illegal drugs before testing.

C) Incorrect. Beta blockers are used to enhance concentration and steady the hands.

D) Incorrect. TNF-a inhibitors are immunosuppressants used to treat inflammatory diseases.

26.

A) Incorrect. There are selenoproteins in the thyroid gland, but thyroid hormone does not contain selenium.

B) **Correct.** Iodine is a component of thyroid hormone, which regulates metabolic rate.

C) Incorrect. Magnesium is not a component of thyroid hormone.

D) Incorrect. Cobalt is not a component of thyroid hormone.

27.

A) Incorrect. Lactic acid does not cause DOMS.

B) Incorrect. Static stretching does not cause DOMS.

C) **Correct.** Micro-tears in the muscle fibers from resistance training cause DOMS.

D) Incorrect. Fit individuals can also experience DOMS.

28.

A) Incorrect. This is the amount of fat kcal, not grams.

B) **Correct.** 2,000 kcal × 0.10 × 1 gram/9 kcal = 22 grams.

C) Incorrect. Fat has 9 kcal per gram, not 10 kcal per gram.

D) Incorrect. This is far less saturated fat than the maximum recommendation.

29. A) **Correct.** Oatmeal, fruits, and beans are sources of soluble fiber.

B) Incorrect. Only plant foods contain fiber.

C) Incorrect. Whole wheat, brown rice, and seeds are sources of insoluble fiber.

D) Incorrect. Vegetable oils contain only fats.

30. A) **Correct.** Measurements over 40 inches for men and 35 inches for women are considered unhealthy.

B) Incorrect. The measurements vary by sex.

C) Incorrect. These thresholds are too high.

D) Incorrect. The measurements vary by sex.

31. A) **Correct.** This is the definition of Golgi tendon organs.

B) Incorrect. While this is a proprioceptor, it is not the correct proprioceptor.

C) Incorrect. This is not a proprioceptor.

D) Incorrect. This is not a proprioceptor.

32. A) Incorrect. This position describes the term dorsal (posterior).

B) **Correct.** Both terms mean toward the front.

C) Incorrect. This is referring to medial.

D) Incorrect. This is referring to distal.

33. A) Incorrect. Marathoners benefit more from slow-twitch muscle fibers.

B) Incorrect. Such swimmers benefit more from slow-twitch muscle fibers.

C) **Correct.** Olympic sprinters require fast-twitch muscle fibers for improved performance.

D) Incorrect. Cross-country cyclists benefit more from slow-twitch muscle fibers.

34. A) **Correct.** Slow-twitch muscle fibers contain more mitochondria than fast-twitch muscle fibers.

B) Incorrect. Fast-twitch muscle fibers have a higher anaerobic capacity.

C) Incorrect. Fast-twitch muscle fibers have a higher force production capability.

D) Incorrect. Slow-twitch muscle fibers are referred to as type I, whereas fast-twitch muscle fibers are categorized into type IIa or IIb.

35. A) Incorrect. Knee flexion is incorrect.

B) **Correct.** These are the two actions of the quadriceps muscles.

C) Incorrect. Knee flexion and hip extension are both incorrect.

D) Incorrect. Hip extension is incorrect.

36. A) Incorrect. This is the wrong phase.

B) **Correct.** This refers to the contraction phase in muscle.

C) Incorrect. This is the wrong phase.

D) Incorrect. Although this is a portion of muscular contraction, it is not a phase during the neuromuscular stimulation process.

37. A) Incorrect. This plane of motion is not correct.

B) Incorrect. This plane of motion is not correct.

C) **Correct.** The elbow extends in the sagittal plane by the contraction of the triceps.

D) Incorrect. This plane of motion is not correct.

38. A) Incorrect. This is the opposite muscle action of the gastrocnemius and is performed by a different muscle group.

B) Incorrect. This is the wrong terminology for the muscular action of the gastrocnemius.

C) **Correct.** This is the action of the gastrocnemius.

D) Incorrect. This is the wrong terminology for the muscular action of the gastrocnemius.

39. A) Incorrect. This is the wrong type of muscle contraction.

B) Incorrect. This is the wrong type of muscle contraction.

C) Incorrect. This is the wrong type of muscle contraction.

D) Correct. This is the definition of isometric muscle contraction.

40. A) Incorrect. This is an increase in joint angle by muscular contraction.

B) Incorrect. This is a combination of many joint movements.

C) Correct. This definition refers to flexion.

D) Incorrect. This is when a joint moves in a circular pattern around an axis.

41. A) Incorrect. The latissimus dorsi is a prime mover in this exercise.

B) Correct. The gluteus medius stabilizes the hip joint during the box step-up.

C) Incorrect. The biceps brachii is a prime mover in this exercise.

D) Incorrect. The quadriceps are a prime mover in this exercise.

42. A) Incorrect. Organs are a collection of tissues.

B) Incorrect. This is an anatomical direction.

C) Incorrect. Organ systems are the next-largest on the biological hierarchy.

D) Correct. This definition refers to organs.

43. **A) Correct.** This is the definition of length-tension relationship.

B) Incorrect. This is the working of two muscle groups to perform the same joint movement.

C) Incorrect. This theory states the crossbridging of actin and myosin for muscle contraction.

D) Incorrect. This is the way in which muscle fibers are recruited with different exercise intensity.

44. A) Incorrect. This refers to hyperplasia.

B) **Correct.** This is the definition of muscular hypertrophy.

C) Incorrect. This refers to muscular atrophy.

D) Incorrect. This is not the definition of muscular hypertrophy.

45. A) **Correct.** These veins collect deoxygenated blood from the body and feed it into the right atrium.

B) Incorrect. The carotid artery feeds oxygenated blood to the head and face.

C) Incorrect. The aorta feeds oxygenated blood to much of the body.

D) Incorrect. The lungs are where deoxygenated blood goes for gas exchange after it exits the right ventricle.

46. A) Incorrect. Rock climbing does not necessarily increase the risk of medial knee injuries in female athletes.

B) Correct. Jumping increases the risk of medial knee injuries in female athletes with increased Q-angles.

C) Incorrect. Ice hockey does not necessarily increase the risk of medial knee injuries in female athletes.

D) Incorrect. Snowboarding does not necessarily increase the risk of medial knee injuries in female athletes.

47. A) Incorrect. This refers to proximal.

B) Incorrect. This refers to superior.

C) Correct. This is the definition of distal.

D) Incorrect. This refers to medial.

48. **A) Correct.** Air travels from the trachea to the bronchi.

B) Incorrect. The mouth is before the trachea.

C) Incorrect. Air flows from the bronchi to the bronchioles.

D) Incorrect. Air flows from the bronchioles to the alveoli for gas exchange.

49. A) Incorrect. The red blood cells carry oxygen to the tissues.

B) **Correct.** The platelets found in blood aid in clotting.

C) Incorrect. White blood cells aid in fighting infection.

D) Incorrect. Water helps blood viscous move through the circulatory system.

50. A) Incorrect. This is not the function of the abdominals.

B) Incorrect. This is not the function of the pectoralis major.

C) Incorrect. This is not the function of the pectoralis minor.

D) **Correct.** The diaphragm helps create a pressure differential in the lungs to aid in respiration.

51. A) Incorrect. This digestion location comes after the esophagus.

B) Incorrect. This digestion location comes after the mouth.

C) **Correct.** Digestion begins in the mouth.

D) Incorrect. This digestion location comes after the stomach.

52. A) Incorrect. The nerves are part of the peripheral nervous system.

B) **Correct.** The central nervous system is made up of the brain and spinal cord.

C) Incorrect. The proprioceptors are found in the muscles.

D) Incorrect. The nerves are part of the peripheral nervous system.

53. A) Incorrect. This occurs when a limb is pulled away from the midline of the body.

B) Incorrect. This occurs as a joint angle increases with muscle contraction.

C) Incorrect. This occurs as the hand is rotated so the palm faces toward the ground.

D) **Correct.** This muscular action refers to adduction.

54. A) Incorrect. This refers to Alzheimer's disease.

B) Incorrect. This refers to osteoporosis.

C) **Correct.** Multiple sclerosis affects the myelin sheaths on axons.

D) Incorrect. Multiple sclerosis affects the myelin sheaths rather than the nucleus.

55. A) Incorrect. This is the process by which the body recruits more motor units to perform the same task.

B) Incorrect. This occurs after several weeks of resistance training.

C) **Correct.** This is the definition of summation.

D) Incorrect. This refers to a single environmental stressor.

56. **A)** **Correct.** Abnormal or disordered heart rhythms are known as arrhythmias.

B) Incorrect. This is part of the female athlete triad.

C) Incorrect. This is abnormally high blood pressure.

D) Incorrect. This is a hardening of the arteries.

57. A) Incorrect. Testosterone is a type of anabolic hormone.

B) Incorrect. IGF is a type of anabolic hormone.

C) Incorrect. Epinephrine is a type of hormone associated with environmental stressors.

D) **Correct.** The two hormone types associated with exercise are anabolic and catabolic.

58. A) Incorrect. Hormones are what an organ secretes, but they are not the organ itself.

B) Incorrect. The brain contains glands, but it is not a gland itself.

C) Incorrect. This is a hormone that is secreted by a gland.

D) **Correct.** This is the definition of a gland.

59. **A)** **Correct.** The hypothalamus controls the autonomic nervous system and the connection of the central nervous and endocrine systems.

B) Incorrect. The hypothalamus does not control the peripheral nervous system and associated nerves.

C) Incorrect. The musculoskeletal system and voluntary skeletal muscle is not controlled by the hypothalamus.

D) Incorrect. This is regulated by the pituitary gland.

60. A) Incorrect. This is the female reproductive organ, but it does not carry these responsibilities.

B) **Correct.** The placenta is an organ that nourishes the fetus during pregnancy.

C) Incorrect. This is the male reproductive organ.

D) Incorrect. This is found in the brain and is responsible for the release of melatonin for sleep regulation.

61. A) Incorrect. The muscles apply force during an isometric movement, and this would be indicated on a force-time curve.

B) Incorrect. This would indicate force being applied quickly but not held isometrically—for example, a single vertical jump.

C) **Correct.** The force-time curve would indicate an increase and then a stabilization of force.

D) Incorrect. This would indicate an exercise where a high force is applied and followed by a lower force isometric movement. For example, a jump with a static hold at the bottom.

62. A) Incorrect. The BMI formula takes height into account.

B) Incorrect. The BMI formula takes height into account.

C) **Correct.** Strength training builds lean muscle mass, which is a healthy kind of excess weight.

D) Incorrect. For a sedentary individual, excess weight would likely be unhealthy fat, and BMI would be a measure of that.

63. A) Incorrect. The resistance and the weight are the same thing.

B) Incorrect. The muscles and the force are the same thing.

C) Incorrect. The resistance and the weight are the same thing.

D) **Correct.** A lever system is comprised of the fulcrum, the resistance, and the force.

64. A) Incorrect. This is the least common type of lever on the body.

B) Incorrect. The body uses all three types of lever systems.

C) Incorrect. This is not the most common type of lever system on the body.

D) **Correct.** This is the most common type of lever system the human body uses.

65. A) Incorrect. This is not Newton's second law of motion.

B) **Correct.** Newton's second law of motion states that force = mass × acceleration.

C) Incorrect. This statement is false.

D) Incorrect. This statement is false.

66. A) Incorrect. This is the amount of work being done by the muscles (work) at a joint divided by the rate at which they are applied (time).

B) Incorrect. This is the rate at which a muscle produces movement through full range of motion at a joint.

C) **Correct.** This is the definition of rotational work.

D) Incorrect. Momentum is the mass of an object times the velocity at which it is traveling.

67. **A)** **Correct.** This is the definition of the lactate threshold.

B) Incorrect. This is the aerobic process of creating ATP for energy.

C) Incorrect. This is the energy system utilized by the body for high-intensity short duration exercise of ten seconds or less.

D) Incorrect. This refers to the body's ability to use either creatine phosphate or muscle glycogen for energy production during exercise.

68. A) Incorrect. This is not a significant exercise expenditure.

B) Incorrect. This caloric expenditure through exercise leaves a 2,500 kcal deficit to be obtained through diet, which could be difficult to maintain.

C) Incorrect. This is a bit less than the optimum caloric expenditure through exercise.

D) Correct. A caloric expenditure of at least 2,000 kcal/week in exercise, combined with a dietary caloric deficit of at least 1,500 kcal/week is recommended to lose at least a pound per week. A sustainable weight loss target is 1 – 2 lb./week.

69. A) Incorrect. There will likely be variations in the distribution of muscle mass between athletes.

B) Incorrect. The two may not have a difference in abdominal muscle strength as both sports require strong abdominal muscles.

C) Correct. The figure skater will likely have more lower body muscle mass as this is the primary mode of movement in this sport.

D) Incorrect. The rock climber will likely have more upper body muscle mass as this is the primary mode of movement in this sport.

70. A) Incorrect. This is the RDA for sedentary nonvegetarians. Active individuals require more protein.

B) Incorrect. An excess of 1.7 g/kg has not been shown to have any performance advantage, regardless of the type of exercise.

C) Incorrect. Protein recommendations vary with activity.

D) Correct. The protein recommendations for each of these categories of people is: 0.8 g/kg (meat eaters) – 0.9 g/kg (vegetarians) for sedentary individuals, 1.2 – 1.4 g/kg for those engaging regularly in endurance activities, and 1.6 – 1.7 g/kg for strength trainers.

71. A) Incorrect. Lean body mass also includes bone, tissues, and organs.

B) Incorrect. Lean body mass contains significant water.

C) Incorrect. The brain contains a lot of fat and contributes to fat mass.

D) Correct. The brain and spinal cord are part of lean body mass but not fat-free mass.

72. A) Incorrect. Muscle growth is incorrect.

B) Incorrect. Fatigue is incorrect.

C) Incorrect. Fatigue is incorrect.

D) Correct. These are the three components of the female athlete triad.

73. A) Correct. This is the function of IGF-1 as a neuroendocrine response to high-intensity exercise.

B) Incorrect. This is the function of catecholamine.

C) Incorrect. This is the function of testosterone.

D) Incorrect. This is the function of catecholamine.

74. A) Incorrect. Hyaline is a type of cartilage.

B) Incorrect. Fibrocartilage is a type of cartilage.

C) Incorrect. Elastic is a type of cartilage.

D) Correct. Ligaments are not a type of cartilage.

75. A) Correct. Children tend to have difficulty regulating body temperature.

B) Incorrect. This is not a common issue among all women.

C) Incorrect. This is not a common issue among older adults.

D) Incorrect. This is not a common issue among men.

76. A) Correct. Disordered eating is one of the components of the female athlete triad and can lead to the other two components: reduced bone mineral density and loss of menstrual cycle.

B) Incorrect. Disordered eating does not lead to improved health.

C) Incorrect. Disordered eating can negatively affect muscle mass development.

D) Incorrect. Disordered eating does not help improve fitness performance.

77. A) Incorrect. This is the job of the digestive system.

B) Incorrect. The bones create red blood cells, but not the muscles.

C) Correct. The levers of the musculoskeletal system are used for human movement.

D) Incorrect. This is the job of the nervous system.

78. A) Incorrect. Cardiac output can be the same at various ages depending on training status and stroke volume of an individual.

B) Incorrect. Age does not necessarily affect blood pressure; younger individuals can have hypertension, and older individuals can have normal values of blood pressure.

C) Correct. Age decreases maximum heart rate.

D) Incorrect. Age does not necessarily affect resting heart rate.

79. A) Correct. Twenty amino acids make up proteins.

B) Incorrect. Eight to ten amino acids are considered essential to the diet, but several more can be synthesized by the body and are the building blocks of proteins.

C) Incorrect. Eight to ten amino acids are considered essential to the diet, but several more can be synthesized by the body and are the building blocks of proteins.

D) Incorrect. Taurine is an additional amino acid to the standard twenty; it is present in the body but is not incorporated into protein.

80. A) Incorrect. The size of the mineral atom has nothing to do with the naming.

B) Correct. Macrominerals are typically present in the body in larger quantities and have larger dietary requirements.

C) Incorrect. Macrominerals do not bind together.

D) Incorrect. Minerals are obtained from the diet.

81. A) Incorrect. Vitamin E is an antioxidant that protects membrane lipids from oxidation.

B) Incorrect. Vitamin C is an antioxidant that protects against free radicals formed from aerobic metabolism.

C) Incorrect. Beta-carotene is a weak antioxidant.

D) Correct. Vitamin K is involved in blood clotting and bone formation. Vitamins E, C, and beta-carotene are antioxidants, although beta-carotene is a relatively weak antioxidant.

82. A) Incorrect. The biceps brachii is a fusiform muscle.

B) Incorrect. The extensor digitorum longus is a unipennate muscle.

C) Incorrect. The rectus abdominis is a parallel muscle.

D) Correct. The pectoralis major is a convergent muscle.

83. A) Incorrect. Thiamine plays no role in anemia.

B) Correct. Folate and vitamin B-12 are critical to the synthesis of nucleotides, which are the building blocks of DNA. When DNA synthesis is impaired, red blood cells cannot divide fast enough and instead grow large.

C) Incorrect. The type of anemia caused by iron deficiency is characterized by a lack of hemoglobin, which is needed to carry sufficient oxygen.

D) Incorrect. Copper deficiency can lead to iron-deficiency anemia because it is involved in iron transport, not megaloblastic anemia.

84. A) Incorrect. The lengthy aerobic demands as well as increased sweat losses associated with endurance exercise are more likely to cause an iron deficiency than strength training.

B) Incorrect. Male athletes are at lower risk than female athletes for iron deficiency since they tend to eat more meat and do not have menstrual iron losses.

C) Incorrect. As described in answer choice A, strength athletes are not at a high risk for iron-deficiency anemia.

D) Correct. Endurance athletes have higher iron requirements as well as higher iron losses. Female athletes have menstrual losses and also tend to consume less calories and meat than males; these can contribute to iron-deficiency anemia. Since iron from meat is the most bioavailable form, vegetarians are also at risk for iron-deficiency anemia, especially vegetarian endurance athletes.

85. A) Incorrect. These devices do not burn significant calories.

B) Incorrect. It is not possible to target specific body areas for fat loss; fat loss with exercise is distributed throughout body fat stores.

C) Incorrect. These devices do not produce significant weight loss.

D) Correct. These devices do not burn fat, and specific areas cannot be targeted effectively for fat loss.

86. **A) Correct.** Carbohydrates in the form of muscle glycogen and possibly liver glycogen, along with blood glucose, muscle triglycerides, blood fatty acids, and lipoproteins are the major fuels for exercise.

B) Incorrect. Although protein can provide fuel for exercise, its contribution is minor compared to that of carbohydrates and fat.

C) Incorrect. Contributions from protein to fuel exercise are minor compared to the contributions made by carbohydrates.

D) Incorrect. The contributions proteins make to fueling exercise are minor; carbohydrates and fat are the main fuels for exercise.

87. A) Incorrect. The glycemic index is more specific than energy density.

B) Incorrect. The glycemic index has nothing to do with glycogen depletion during exercise.

C) Correct. The glycemic index is the area under the blood glucose curve (AUC) over a two-hour time period following ingestion of the food, divided by the AUC of a standard food (usually white bread) times 100.

D) Incorrect. There are factors other than just the percentage of carbohydrates that affect blood glucose response to a food, such as the type of carbohydrate and the amount of fiber in the food.

88. A. Incorrect. While sodium is responsible for the transmission of electrical signals across nerve and muscle cell membranes, chloride is not.

B. Incorrect. While potassium is responsible for the transmission of electrical signals across nerve and muscle cell membranes, chloride is not.

C) Correct. The changes in membrane potentials that transmit electrical signals are caused by the flow of sodium and potassium ions across the membrane.

D. Incorrect. While sodium is responsible for the transmission of electrical signals across nerve and muscle cell membranes, magnesium is not.

89. A) Incorrect. These are the smaller heart chambers.

B) Correct. The ventricles are the larger heart chambers.

C) Incorrect. These carry deoxygenated blood to the heart.

D) Incorrect. These separate the chambers of the heart.

90. A) Incorrect. The word creation is incorrect.

B) Correct. This is the correct acronym.

C) Incorrect. The word extreme is incorrect.

D) Incorrect. The word pre-exercise is incorrect.

91. **A)** **Correct.** To maintain hydration, it is recommended to consume 20 – 36 oz. of fluid, preferably a sport drink with electrolytes, and ideally spread out at 15 – 20 minute intervals.

B) Incorrect. A fluid intake of 8 – 12 oz. per hour is not enough to maintain hydration during periods of prolonged exercise.

C) Incorrect. A fluid intake of 10 – 15 oz. per hour is not enough to maintain hydration during prolonged exercise.

D) Incorrect. It would be difficult to consume 40 – 45 oz. of fluid per hour, and such a quantity is more than necessary to maintain hydration.

92. **A)** Incorrect. Body composition does not divide out carbohydrates, protein, or water.

B) **Correct.** Body composition refers to the relative percentage of fat versus everything else: muscle, soft tissues, organs, and bone.

C) Incorrect. Both bone and soft tissues contribute to fat-free mass.

D) Incorrect. There is water associated with both the fat mass and fat-free mass.

93. **A)** Incorrect. Saliva primarily helps break down food in the mouth.

B) **Correct.** This is the function of saliva.

C) Incorrect. Nutrient absorption primarily occurs in the small intestine.

D) Incorrect. Water absorption primarily occurs in the large intestine.

94. **A)** **Correct.** The myelin sheath helps speed up nervous transmission of electrical impulses.

B) Incorrect. Impulses travel away from the dendrites (and soma) along the axon on a neuron.

C) Incorrect. The myelin sheaths do not protect against multiple sclerosis; they are damaged by it.

D) Incorrect. The myelin sheaths do not prevent Alzheimer's disease, and there is no known cure.

95. **A)** Incorrect. Sleep deprivation can lead to overeating and poor food choices.

B) Incorrect. In type 2 diabetes, tissues are less responsive to the stimulation of glucose uptake by insulin, which leads to high blood glucose. Taking insulin to treat diabetes can also stimulate the storage of glucose as fat. Exercise can help burn excess glucose, lowering the need for insulin and helping to prevent weight gain.

C) Incorrect. Certain antidepressants tend to cause weight gain.

D) **Correct.** The drug metformin is used to increase insulin sensitivity and decrease glucose production by the liver in type 2 diabetics. It does not lead to weight gain and may assist somewhat in weight loss.

PRACTICE TEST ONE PRACTICAL/APPLIED ANSWER KEY

1.
   A) Incorrect. The Rockport walk test assesses cardiorespiratory endurance.

   B) Incorrect. The push-up test is a muscular endurance test.

   C) Correct. The hexagon test is used to assess speed, agility, and quickness.

   D) Incorrect. The twelve-minute run test is used to assess cardiorespiratory endurance.

2.
   A) Incorrect. With female clients, the thigh is measured, but the biceps and chest are not.

   B) Correct. The triceps, suprailium, and thigh are the three sites measured on female clients.

   C) Incorrect. The thigh and suprailium are measured, but the subscapular is not measured on female clients.

   D) Incorrect. The suprailium and thigh are measured on female clients; the biceps are not.

3.
   A) Correct. The 300-yard shuttle test is used to measure anaerobic capacity.

   B) Incorrect. The LEFT is used to measure agility in the sagittal and frontal plane.

   C) Incorrect. The pro-agility test measures lateral speed and agility.

   D) Incorrect. The t-test is used to assess overall agility while moving forward, laterally, and backward.

4.
   A) Incorrect. Short-distance sprints will help football players since the longest distance they run is one hundred yards.

   B) Correct. Long-distance running does not follow the principle of specificity when it comes to football.

   C) Incorrect. Power exercises that develop speed will improve football players' one-hundred-yard yard sprint time.

   D) Incorrect. Muscular endurance exercises will help to benefit short-distance sprints.

5.
   A) Incorrect. A mesocycle typically includes multiple microcycles.

   B) Incorrect. A macrocycle includes the entire periodization.

   C) Correct. A microcycle is the shortest cycle in a periodization.

   D) Incorrect. The preparatory period typically involves mesocycles and microcycles.

6.
   A) Incorrect. A flexibility assessment is generally included in a fitness assessment.

   B) Incorrect. A static postural assessment is generally included in a fitness assessment.

   C) Correct. An assessment of daily caloric intake is generally not included during a fitness assessment.

   D) Incorrect. A cardiorespiratory capacity assessment is generally not included in a fitness assessment.

7.
   A) Incorrect. Movement assessments do not test maximal force.

   B) Incorrect. Movement assessments do not test core strength.

   C) Incorrect. Movement assessments do not test agility and speed.

   D) Correct. Movement assessments are used to test dynamic posture.

8.
   A) Incorrect. Certification through leading organizations does not guarantee more money.

   B) Correct. Clients who are thorough will research a fitness professional to make sure he or she has expertise in the field.

   C) Incorrect. Certifications cannot guarantee client results.

   D) Incorrect. Fitness certifications are not necessarily proof of higher education or training, although certified professionals have often obtained both.

9.
   A) Incorrect. Twenty seconds is shorter than the recommended time.

   B) Incorrect. Sixty seconds is longer than the recommended time.

C) **Correct.** Thirty seconds is the recommended time for static stretching.

D) Incorrect. Ten seconds is shorter than the recommended time.

10. A) Incorrect. Hypertension refers to high blood pressure.

B) Incorrect. Hyperventilation is an increased respiration rate.

C) Incorrect. Delayed onset muscle soreness is the normal physiological response related to micro-tears in the muscle fibers, causing acute muscular soreness.

D) **Correct.** The definition provided describes overtraining.

11. A) Incorrect. The legal parameters are not called scope of product.

B) Incorrect. Legality of specialization is not the proper name for the legal parameters.

C) **Correct.** Scope of practice is the term that describes the legal parameters within which credentialed or licensed health professionals must work.

D) Incorrect. Terms of work is not the proper name.

12. **A)** **Correct.** This network is called the allied healthcare continuum.

B) Incorrect. The term training continuum describes a progressive system in exercise technique.

C) Incorrect. While those in the network are considered health professionals, this is not the proper name of the network.

D) Incorrect. The term health maintenance professionals is not correct.

13. A) Incorrect. The bench press test would not be appropriate for this goal.

B) Incorrect. The hexagon test would not be appropriate for this goal.

C) **Correct.** The Rockport walk test would be the most appropriate test for the goal of lowering a client's blood pressure.

D) Incorrect. The three-hundred-yard shuttle test would not be appropriate for this goal.

14. **A)** **Correct.** A trainer should tell a client complaining of pain to visit his or her physician.

B) Incorrect. A trainer should not refer a client to see a friend.

C) Incorrect. A trainer should not refer this client to a massage therapist because the trainer does not know the scope of the injury or why the pain is occurring.

D) Incorrect. A trainer should always express interest in helping a client relieve his or her pain.

15. A) Incorrect. Error points are given for this deviation.

B) **Correct.** This is not a deviation.

C) Incorrect. Error points are given for this deviation.

D) Incorrect. Error points are given for this deviation.

16. A) Incorrect. Core exercises typically recruit large muscle groups and have multiple joint motions.

B) Incorrect. Open kinetic chain exercises do activate smaller muscle groups, but they are not used for just rehabilitative purposes.

C) Incorrect. PNF stretching is stretching used for rehabilitative purposes and typically requires assistance from another person.

D) **Correct.** Assistance exercises are used for rehabilitative purposes; they isolate a specific, smaller muscle group.

17. A) Incorrect. Questions pertaining to a client's sleep patterns should be included on a lifestyle questionnaire.

B) Incorrect. Questions pertaining to a client's stressors should be included on a lifestyle questionnaire.

C) **Correct.** Questions pertaining to a client's friends are not necessary on a lifestyle questionnaire.

D) Incorrect. Questions pertaining to a client's smoking habits should be included on a lifestyle questionnaire.

18. A) Incorrect. Arthritis typically causes INCREASED joint pain.

B) Incorrect. Arthritis will not necessarily affect the motivation level of the client.

C) Correct. Joint range of motion can be decreased due to arthritis.

D) Incorrect. Muscular atrophy typically increases around an arthritic joint.

19. A) Incorrect. Nurses are part of the AHC.

B) Incorrect. Psychologists are part of the AHC.

C) Incorrect. Occupational therapists are part of the AHC.

D) Correct. Psychics are not part of the AHC.

20. A) Incorrect. The long jump test is used to assess horizontal bilateral power.

B) Incorrect. The Margaria-Kalamen test is used to assess lower body power.

C) Correct. The star excursion test is used to assess dynamic balance.

D) Incorrect. The reactive strength index is used to assess the body's ability to perform plyometric activities.

21. A) Incorrect. A professional trainer would NOT wear khaki pants or jeans.

B) Correct. Tasteful athletic attire is appropriate for a professional trainer.

C) Incorrect. Revealing athletic attire is NOT appropriate for a professional trainer to wear.

D) Incorrect. Strong cologne or perfume is NOT appropriate for a professional trainer.

22. A) Incorrect. The handheld bioelectrical impedance device is used to measure body fat.

B) Correct. The sphygmomanometer is used to assess blood pressure.

C) Incorrect. Calipers are used to assess body fat percentage.

D) Incorrect. The scale is used to measure weight.

23. A) Incorrect. The client should be seated slightly upright.

B) Incorrect. Range of motion may be reduced by the client's physical changes; however, it does not need to be reduced dramatically.

C) Incorrect. Abdominal exercises should be encouraged for pregnant clients.

D) Correct. The client should be seated slightly upright.

24. A) Incorrect. The second transition is a recovery period.

B) Incorrect. Sports-specific training occurs during the other three periods.

C) Incorrect. The athlete should still participate in physical activity in the second transition period.

D) Correct. The second transition period should involve active rest that includes non-specific recreational activities not related to the athlete's competition.

25. **A) Correct.** This test measures one's ability to change directions and stabilize the body at high speeds.

B) Incorrect. This test measures an individual's agility while moving laterally, forward, and backward.

C) Incorrect. This test measures lateral speed and agility.

D) Incorrect. This test is used to measure total body bilateral power.

26. A) Incorrect. This is not a subcategory of core exercises.

B) Incorrect. This is the main classification of core exercises, not a subcategory.

C) Correct. Power exercises use multiple muscle groups and joint motions, but are not load-bearing, like structural.

D) Incorrect. This is a form of stretching.

27. A) Incorrect. Static stretching is a technique that uses an implement to hold the leg in place.

B)   Incorrect. Passive stretching is not a cardio warm-up.

C)   Correct. Dynamic stretching includes stretches that are more intense and utilize full range of motion, so when they are performed in a circuit, they could be a challenging cardio warm-up.

D)   Incorrect. Active stretching is indeed a type of stretching that uses slow and controlled movements to increase range of motion, but it would not be challenging for a cardio warm-up.

28. A)   Incorrect. General warm-up and SMR should come before static stretching.

B)   Incorrect. Dynamic stretching should be after static stretching.

C)   Incorrect. Cardio warm-up should come before static stretching.

D)   Correct. SMR is ideal to do before static stretching to ensure the loosening of muscle knots.

29. A)   Incorrect. This is the definition of a pyramid set.

B)   Incorrect. This is the definition of a multiple set program.

C)   Correct. This is the definition of a superset.

D)   Incorrect. This is the definition of circuit training.

30. A)   Incorrect. The excessive fatigue associated with this volume and load range can negate performance during the season.

B)   Correct. The off-season should include a period of muscular endurance development because athletic performance will not be hindered during competition.

C)   Incorrect. Excessive fatigue from muscular endurance training should be avoided during the competitive period because it can cause deleterious effects on performance.

D)   Incorrect. The second transition period should involve recreational activities and a break from resistance training protocols.

31. A)   Incorrect. A workout is the complete dynamic warm-up, training stimulus, cooldown, and stretching.

B)   Incorrect. The load refers to the amount of weight being lifted in a set.

C)   Incorrect. Overload is the principle that increases to training variables stimulates the muscle to adapt.

D)   Correct. This is the definition of a set.

32. A)   Incorrect. Static stretching should happen in the middle of the warm-up.

B)   Incorrect. PNF stretching should come in the middle of the warm-up, in lieu of static stretching if rehab is needed.

C)   Correct. Dynamic stretching should be done at the end of the warm-up to target the muscle groups that will be worked during a workout.

D)   Incorrect. SMR stretching is done after the general cardio warm-up if needed.

33. **A)   Correct.** A push press is an explosive, standing shoulder press, which is an advanced shoulder press.

B)   Incorrect. While the primary movers are shoulders, the standing upright row is a pulling move, not a pushing move.

C)   Incorrect. The primary movers for a low row are the latissimus dorsi and the erector spinae.

D)   Incorrect. The primary mover for the push-up is the pectorals.

34. A)   Incorrect. Spotting requires at least one person.

B)   Incorrect. A dumbbell shoulder press requires one spotter.

C)   Incorrect. A dumbbell shoulder press requires one spotter.

D)   Correct. One spotter is required behind the lifter, supporting the wrists.

35. A)   Incorrect. The client may not know the signs and symptoms of overtraining, or may give an inaccurate response.

B)   Incorrect. The client's relatives may not know the signs and symptoms of overtraining.

C) **Correct.** Keeping accurate records of the client's progress means the trainer can consult data to determine whether the client is overtraining. There are often physiological and psychological symptoms associated with overtraining.

D) Incorrect. Another fitness professional meeting the client for the first time might consider the client's abilities normal.

36. A) Incorrect. Relativity refers to a theory in physics.

B) Incorrect. Honesty refers to the principle of personal values.

C) **Correct.** This term describes the degree to which a test or test item measures what is supposed to be measured.

D) Incorrect. This is part of an assessment.

37. A) Incorrect. Static stretching should not be part of the warm-up.

B) Incorrect. Single-muscle group exercises and plyometrics should not be performed until after the warm-up is complete.

C) **Correct.** These three items should always be included in the warm-up process for ideal preparation.

D) Incorrect. Although dynamic stretching and foam rolling may be beneficial to the field hockey player, PNF stretching may inhibit the player's performance during the workout.

38. A) Incorrect. The Golgi tendon organ is in the muscle spindles.

B) **Correct.** The Golgi tendon organ is the primary stimulator in autogenic inhibition.

C) Incorrect. The tendons are not in the muscles; they are connectors between the muscles and bones.

D) Incorrect. Ligaments are tissues that connect bones to each other.

39. A) Incorrect. This rest period is too short.

B) Incorrect. This rest period is too short.

C) Incorrect. This rest period is too short.

D) **Correct.** Heavier loads require longer rest periods, and 90 percent of 1RM requires a full three-minute rest period for adequate recovery.

40. A) Incorrect. A stretching partner is used in PNF stretching.

B) Incorrect. Active stretching uses bodyweight only.

C) Incorrect. Boxes and medicine balls are used for power training.

D) **Correct.** SMR utilizes gravity and a foam roller to ease muscle tension.

41. A) Incorrect. Nodding indicates positive body language.

B) Incorrect. Leaning forward is another way to indicate a positive body language.

C) **Correct.** Wringing hands is a negative body language indicator.

D) Incorrect. A firm handshake also indicates positive body language.

42. A) Incorrect. This should not be the main focus of a resistance training program for children and adolescents.

B) Incorrect. Specific and repetitive movements can cause overuse injuries even in children.

C) Incorrect. High-intensity exercise may be part of the sport they participate in, but technique and form are more important in their training programs.

D) **Correct.** Proper technique and form development should be the goal of child and adolescent resistance training programs.

43. A) Incorrect. A spotter cannot be used in a hip hinge motion.

B) Incorrect. Medicine ball slams are explosive exercises and therefore cannot use a spotter; the weight is not heavy enough.

C) **Correct.** Back-loaded squats can use up to three spotters to ensure proper form.

D) Incorrect. Walking lunges are characterized by forward motion and cannot use a spotter.

44. A) Incorrect. Enthusiasm is the only one of the three attributes described correctly.

B) Correct. Confidence, enthusiasm, and professionalism are the three attributes a trainer should personify when meeting with a client.

C) Incorrect. Confidence is the only one of the three attributes described correctly.

D) Incorrect. None of these are among the three attributes described in the text.

45. A) Incorrect. The DEXA scan is used to measure body fat percentage.

B) Correct. Body mass index measurements do not measure body fat but determine if an individual's weight is appropriate for his or her height.

C) Incorrect. Near-infrared interactance is used to measure body fat percentage.

D) Incorrect. Air displacement plethysmography is used to measure body fat percentage.

46. A) Incorrect. The palms are facing up on a supinated grip.

B) Incorrect. In an alternating grip, one palm is up and the other is down.

C) Incorrect. In a false grip, the palms facing are down.

D) Correct. The palms are facing each other in a neutral grip.

47. A) Incorrect. A heart rate taken before a workout would be considered a preworkout heart rate.

B) Incorrect. A heart rate taken at the end of the day may be affected by factors such as stress, food, or beverages consumed.

C) Correct. The best time to measure resting heart rate is upon rising in the morning for three consecutive days.

D) Incorrect. Taking heart rate measurements during a workout would alter the heart rate due to the activity level.

48. A) Incorrect. Alternated grips are both underhanded and overhanded.

B) Incorrect. Supinated grips are underhanded.

C) Correct. A pronated grip is also known as an overhanded grip.

D) Incorrect. A clean grip requires wrist flexion: the palms are facing the ceiling and the fingers are supporting a barbell at the shoulders.

49. A) Incorrect. 1:5 allows too long a recovery period to elicit an overload effect for cardiovascular training when the activity is as light as jogging.

B) Incorrect. This ratio may be too difficult for individuals who are just starting.

C) Incorrect. This ratio will likely be too difficult for individuals new to running.

D) Correct. A 1:1 work-to-rest ratio of jogging and walking should be enough for most individuals who are new to running programs.

50. **A) Correct.** Motions from side to side cross the plane that bisects the body into anterior and posterior halves.

B) Incorrect. Motions from front to back cross the plane that bisects the body into left and right haves—the sagittal plane.

C) Incorrect. Twisting motions cross the plane that bisects the body into superior and inferior halves—the transverse plane.

D) Incorrect. This is not a plane of motion.

51. **A) Correct.** A tuck jump is a plyometrics exercise.

B) Incorrect. A tuck jump uses explosive force, but explosive training is not a training classification.

C) Incorrect: A tuck jump is a bodyweight exercise and therefore not considered resistance training.

D) Incorrect: Kettlebells are not used while doing a tuck jump.

52. A) Incorrect. Only the shoulders are a point of contact in a standing or sitting position.

    B) Correct. These are the three parts of the body that should maintain points of contact with the wall or dowel.

    C) Incorrect. The calves are not a point of contact in a standing or sitting position.

    D) Incorrect. The heels are not a point of contact in a standing or sitting position.

53. A) Incorrect. The client can benefit from other modes of aerobic exercise including running.

    B) Incorrect. The client can benefit from other modes of aerobic exercise including these two.

    C) Correct. For general health benefits, the mode of aerobic exercise does not matter and whatever modes the client prefers should be implemented.

    D) Incorrect. For improvements to cardiovascular and respiratory fitness, which are important general health benefits, aerobic exercise is required.

54. A) Incorrect. Another name for a forearm muscle is extensor carpi.

    B) Incorrect. Another name for a thigh muscle is the quadriceps.

    C) Correct. The gastrocnemius is the power producing muscle of the calf.

    D) Incorrect. The trapezius is a stabilizing muscle in the neck.

55. A) Incorrect. Age is a personal attribute.

    B) Correct. Accessibility is an environmental factor.

    C) Incorrect. Time is a personal attribute.

    D) Incorrect. Fitness level is a personal attribute.

56. A) Incorrect. Horizontal loading refers to performing multiple sets of a single exercise with intermittent rest periods.

    B) Incorrect. Single set refers to performing one set of each exercise during a workout.

    C) Incorrect. Interval training refers to using a timer to determine the work-to-rest ratio rather than repetitions.

    D) Correct. Vertical loading is a form of circuit training that loads different muscles per exercise to minimize rest.

57. A) Incorrect. While quickness and agility are connected, agility is the body's ability to accelerate and decelerate more so than reacting to a direction change.

    B) Correct. Quickness is the body's ability to react to changing direction.

    C) Incorrect. Readiness is not a term that describes an exercise function.

    D) Incorrect. Stabilization is the body's ability to utilize the core efficiently.

58. A) Incorrect. The terms power, muscle, and matter do not represent progressive fitness levels.

    B) Incorrect. Hard is not a fitness level.

    C) Correct. The terms stabilization, strength, and power represent three fitness levels.

    D) Incorrect. Body is not correct.

59. A) Incorrect. The drawing-in maneuver does activate the core.

    B) Incorrect. The drawing-in maneuver maintains neutral posturing.

    C) Incorrect. The drawing-in maneuver is used for all core exercises.

    D) Correct. The drawing-in maneuver does not stretch the hips.

60. A) Incorrect. Though plyometrics do increase muscular power, they may place dangerous forces on the already overstressed joints of overweight individuals.

    B) Incorrect. This is an opinion of the client and not relevant to the question.

    C) Incorrect. They are in the category of higher intensity exercises and can be difficult for many people.

    D) Correct. The force from landing after a plyometric jump exercise places excessive stress on the joints of the ankles, knees, and hips, and may be dangerous for individuals who are overweight or obese.

61. A) Incorrect. Seven points of contact is appropriate for a supine position and would include the right calf and left calf.

B) Incorrect. Three points of contact refers to a neutral standing position—the head, mid-back, and glutes would touch the wall.

C) Incorrect. There are no body positions that require four points of contact.

D) Correct. The five points of contact in a semi-supine position are at the head, shoulders, glutes, right foot, and left foot.

62. **A) Correct.** The mode of cardiovascular exercise for weight loss is not important.

B) Incorrect. Variety in cardio activities is beneficial for weight-loss clients because it keeps programs from becoming stale.

C) Incorrect. The mode should vary in the energy systems used to prevent program staleness.

D) Incorrect. If the client is cleared for physical activity and has no restrictions detailed by a physician, the client can participate in cardio that has impact.

63. **A) Correct.** Plyometric moves are compact to aid in footwork focus and aerodynamics.

B) Incorrect. SAQ exercises should be fast, not slow.

C) Incorrect. No exercise should be painful—only challenging.

D) Incorrect. Here, controlled is synonymous with slow.

64. **A) Correct.** Structural exercises load the spine, the main postural component of the body to increase strength.

B) Incorrect. Power exercises are core exercises, but they are not load bearing and typically utilize reactive motions to increase force production.

C) Incorrect. Agility exercises typically do not use any weight and focus on agility through footwork and deceleration.

D) Incorrect. Assistance exercises are not core exercises and recruit single joint action and small muscle groups.

65. A) Incorrect. The waist-to-hip ratio correlates chronic diseases and fat stored in the midsection.

B) Incorrect. Air displacement plethysmography (BOD POD) is used to assess body composition.

C) Correct. Body mass index is used to assess weight relative to height.

D) Incorrect. Skinfold measurements are used to assess body composition.

66. A) Incorrect. Plyometrics training increases force production.

B) Incorrect. Cardio training increases aerobic endurance.

C) Incorrect. Free weight training increases prime mover and joint strength.

D) Correct. Core training increases core strength with balance.

67. **A) Correct.** Ice skaters utilize full range of motion and lateral explosive repetitions.

B) Incorrect. Ice skaters require balance, but the abdominals are not the prime movers, and the repetitions are not slow and steady.

C) Incorrect. This is a bodyweight move.

D) Incorrect. There is no focus on muscle lengthening in ice skaters.

68. **A) Correct.** The 1RM is single repetition maximum to determine the client's maximal effort of strength for one repetition of an exercise.

B) Incorrect. The 1RM determines strength for a single exercise, not all exercises.

C) Incorrect. Target heart rate zone is determined by the Karvonen formula.

D) Incorrect. Although estimates can be made from the 1RM for submaximal efforts, the 1RM test is for a single repetition.

69. A) Incorrect. Sandbags, resistance tubes, and stability balls are used for functional training.

B) Incorrect. Free weights, functional equipment, and weight machines are used for resistance training.

C) Incorrect. Bodyweight, medicine balls, and boxes are used for power training.

D) Correct. Treadmills, elliptical trainers, and rowing machines are used for aerobic training.

70. A) Incorrect. Push jerks are explosive moves, while structural exercises are controlled.

B) Incorrect. Stability exercises focus on core strength and controlled repetitions.

C) Correct. Push jerks incorporate multiple muscle groups and challenge force production while building strength through explosive motions.

D) Incorrect. While the lifter is standing, this does not classify any exercise; it is too generalized.

71. **A) Correct.** Detraining occurs more rapidly in the aspects of a cardiovascular training program.

B) Incorrect. There is a more gradual detraining in muscular strength and some is retained following a short period of exercise cessation.

C) Incorrect. Previously trained clients will retain some of their strength following cessation of a training program.

D) Incorrect. This will depend on the type of professional athlete, and any muscular strength training will be retained slightly.

72. A) Incorrect. Cardiorespiratory assessments are used to help personal trainers identify safe and effective exercise intensities for cardiorespiratory exercise.

B) Incorrect. Movement assessments are used to observe dynamic posture.

C) Incorrect. Muscular endurance assessments are used to determine muscular endurance capacity.

D) Correct. Physiological assessments, such as resting heart rate and blood pressure measurements, are indicators of an individual's general fitness and overall health.

73. A) Incorrect. Push-and-pull routines use a variety of large muscle groups on opposing sides of the body, limiting the risk of muscular imbalances.

B) Incorrect. The bodyweight training program described includes exercises for both chest and back muscles, reducing the chance of one-dimensional training.

C) Incorrect. A trained yoga instructor will incorporate exercises to increase flexibility and utilize all the major muscle groups, reducing the risk of muscular imbalances.

D) Correct. Unilateral training programs have a high risk of causing muscular imbalances. A program focusing on the chest and anterior deltoids specifically can cause rounding of the shoulders and muscular imbalances of the upper body.

74. A) Incorrect. This is a supinated grip.

B) Correct. The thumb wraps around the same side as the fingers.

C) Incorrect. This is a hook grip.

D) Incorrect. This is the same as a supinated grip.

75. A) Incorrect. Static stretching can limit strength and power output, causing poor performance and potential injury.

B) Incorrect. Static stretching can harm power exercise performance such as plyometrics.

C) Incorrect. Cardiovascular exercise should follow the same warm-up protocol as resistance training.

D) Correct. Static stretching should be implemented in a flexibility program after the muscles have been warmed up and exercised to elongate the muscles.

76. **A)** **Correct.** Typical mesocycles include multiple microcycles and last around six to twelve weeks.

B) Incorrect. This time period is too short.

C) Incorrect. This time period is too long and is more likely for a macrocycle.

D) Incorrect. This time period is far too long for a single mesocycle and the client will never reach peak performance.

77. **A)** Incorrect. The floor crunch lifts the head, neck, and shoulders, while the reverse crunch lifts the hip flexors and the pelvic floor; therefore the floor crunch is not the best regression for the reverse crunch.

B) Incorrect. The floor crunch is performed in the semi-supine position, while the plank hold is performed in the prone position; therefore the floor crunch is not the best regression for the plank hold.

C) Incorrect. The floor crunch lifts the head, neck, and shoulders, while the hip bridge lifts the glutes and the pelvic floor; therefore the floor crunch is not the best regression for the hip bridge.

D) **Correct.** The floor crunch targets the same muscles and follows the same range of motion as the ball crunch; however the floor crunch allows for more stabilization than the ball crunch. Thus it is an ideal regression for a client who is not ready for the controlled instability a stability ball provides.

78. **A)** Incorrect. Using the ABC model of behavior to identify triggers is an example of relapse prevention and recovery plans.

B) **Correct.** Planning a weekly menu and a shopping list is an example of time management, not relapse prevention and recovery plans.

C) Incorrect. Not focusing on fault is an example of relapse prevention and recovery plans.

D) Incorrect. Relapse prevention and recovery plans can include creating contingency plans.

79. **A)** Incorrect. The shoulders reveal upper crossed syndrome.

B) Incorrect. The foot and ankle reveal pronation distortion syndrome.

C) Incorrect. The head and cervical spine reveal upper crossed syndrome.

D) **Correct.** The lumbo/pelvic/hip complex reveals lower crossed syndrome.

80. **A)** Incorrect. An estimated maximum heart rate is used in the formula.

B) **Correct.** The formula is used to calculate the target heart rate for an activity.

C) Incorrect. The client's resting heart rate is used in the formula.

D) Incorrect. Heart rate recovery is determined using another method.

81. **A)** Incorrect. Flexibility is not greatly improved by either of these training techniques.

B) Incorrect. Power exercises are high intensity.

C) Incorrect. Muscular endurance exercises are lower intensity.

D) **Correct.** Since technique is important with power exercises, they should be performed before the muscles suffer from fatigue and performance suffers.

82. **A)** Incorrect. Forward movement speed would be more important for the players moving up and down the field.

B) Incorrect. Steady-state cardiovascular exercise will not benefit either position more.

C) Incorrect. All positions in soccer will benefit from kicking and core power exercises.

D) **Correct.** The lateral movement requirement for the goaltender is higher than for the players and therefore the goaltender will benefit more from specific movements in this plane.

83. **A)** Incorrect. Progression refers to a gradual increase in intensity throughout a training program.

B) Incorrect. Regression refers to a decrease in difficulty of exercise due to limitation or inability to perform the exercise.

C) Incorrect. Detraining is the effect of cessation of a training program.

D) Correct. This is the principle of specificity.

84. A) Incorrect. Two spotters is too few.

B) Correct. There should be room for at least three spotters at a free weight barbell bench.

C) Incorrect. One spotter is not enough for a free weight bench.

D) Incorrect. There must be room for the lifter and at least three spotters.

85. A) Incorrect. The goal is specific in that the client wants to lose twenty-five pounds.

B) Incorrect. The goal is time-stamped in that the client wants to lose the weight in two months.

C) Correct. The goal is not realistic as this much weight loss is dangerous and unsustainable by healthy weight-loss methods.

D) Incorrect. The goal is measurable in that the client's weight is the measurement.

86. A) Incorrect. This amount of training increase is too little to elicit an overload effect and training progression.

B) Correct. The cardiovascular training variables should not be increased by more than 10% from workout to workout.

C) Incorrect. This increase is too much and may cause overtraining.

D) Incorrect. This increase is too much and may cause overtraining.

87. **A) Correct.** Cardiovascular retraining after a period of detraining can take several months to return to peak performance.

B) Incorrect. The body does not recover cardiovascular fitness that quickly.

C) Incorrect. Detraining does have an impact on cardiovascular fitness.

D) Incorrect. With a healthy client, proper program design, and implementation it should not take several years.

88. A) Incorrect. The LPHC should be viewed posteriorly.

B) Correct. These checkpoints should be viewed laterally.

C) Incorrect. The knees should be viewed anteriorly.

D) Incorrect. The ankles and feet should be viewed anteriorly.

89. A) Incorrect. A macrocycle includes off-season training as well.

B) Correct. The macrocycle encompasses the entire training periodization.

C) Incorrect. A macrocycle includes in-season training as well.

D) Incorrect. A macrocycle includes all preparatory, transition, competition, and second transition periods.

90. A) Incorrect. Resistance training effects are retained longer than cardiovascular gains after stopping an exercise program.

B) Correct. Cardiovascular gains are noticeably different only two weeks after training cessation.

C) Incorrect. Gender does not make a significant difference in detraining effects.

D) Incorrect. Gender does not make a significant difference in detraining effects.

91. A) Incorrect. Excessive frequency may not necessarily cause rapid gains because overuse injuries are more likely.

B) Incorrect. Excessive frequency may cause added stress due to the body constantly being stressed through exercise.

C) Incorrect. Training intensity and frequency are two different variables.

D) Correct. Overuse injuries often occur due to excessive training frequency.

92. A) Incorrect. Interval training typically involves work-to-rest ratios and is not long distance.

B) Incorrect. Zone training describes a method for increasing the intensity of aerobic conditioning, starting at long distance and working up to sprints at near-maximum heart rate.

C) Incorrect. Anaerobic endurance is similar to interval training, in which rest periods are required for repeated high-intensity bouts of exercise.

D) Correct. A 10-kilometer row is a steady-state aerobic exercise because a steady heart rate is maintained for the majority of the event, which has a long duration.

93. A) Incorrect. The triceps is a primary mover in a triceps extension.

B) Correct. The forearm is a primary mover for a wrist curl.

C) Incorrect. The shoulder is a primary mover for a lateral raise.

D) Incorrect. The biceps is a synergist muscle for the wrist curl.

94. A) Incorrect. Diet journaling is a self-monitoring tool to modify behavior.

B) Incorrect. Activity tracking is another example of a self-monitoring tool.

C) Correct. This is an example of the rewarding technique for behavior modification.

D) Incorrect. Incorporating weekly weigh-ins would be considered a self-monitoring tool.

95. A) Incorrect. Decrease in weight causes decrease in intensity.

B) Incorrect. Increase in volume causes decrease in weight and therefore decrease in intensity.

C) Correct. Increase in weight causes an increase in intensity.

D) Incorrect. Increase in repetitions is similar to increase in volume, causing a decrease in intensity.

96. A) Incorrect. There are ways to progress a single-leg squat.

B) Incorrect. This would be a regression of the same exercise.

C) Correct. Adding weight to the exercise will increase the intensity and be a progression.

D) Incorrect. A new exercise would not be a progression of the same exercise.

97. A) Incorrect. A one-minute rest period is insufficient for recovery.

B) Incorrect. A rest period of less than thirty seconds is far too short for recovery.

C) Correct. At heavy loads and low volumes, rest periods should be three minutes.

D) Incorrect. Six minutes is too long a recovery period, and the muscles will start to cool down.

98. A) Incorrect. Lower back pain does not require a client to see a medical professional.

B) Incorrect. Anterior knee pain does not require immediate medical attention.

C) Correct. A client who has had a recent complication due to cardiac disease must be referred to a medical professional before the assessment may begin.

D) Incorrect. A client who does not feel well generally does not need an immediate medical referral.

99. A) Incorrect. This is associated with misaligned lumbo/pelvic/hip complex.

B) Correct. This is associated with misaligned neck, shoulders, and midback.

C) Incorrect. This is associated with misalignment of the feet and ankles.

D) Incorrect. This is associated with pronation distortion, causing the knees to internally rotate.

100. A) Incorrect. The program is incomplete and missing warm-up, cooldown, and cardiovascular training.

B) Incorrect. The program is incomplete and missing warm-up, cooldown, and resistance training.

C) Incorrect. The program is incomplete and missing warm-up, cooldown, resistance training, and cardiovascular training.

D) **Correct.** This program includes all of the major components of a workout.

101. A) **Correct.** These forms are used by fitness professionals to ensure they have taken all measures to improve client safety prior to exercise, to inform the client, and to ensure the trainer has the client's consent to begin training.

B) Incorrect. A client's hobbies may help in designing an exercise plan, but they will not minimize risk, and a bloodwork form is beyond the fitness professional's scope of practice.

C) Incorrect. The bloodwork form is beyond the fitness professional's scope of practice.

D) Incorrect. The fitness assessment should not be performed until all forms are completed and signed.

102. A) **Correct.** The resting heart rate is the strongest indicator of how the cardiorespiratory system is responding and adapting to exercise.

B) Incorrect. The 1.5-mile run is an assessment of cardiorespiratory fitness but does not provide a strong indicator of how the cardiorespiratory system responds to exercise.

C) Incorrect. Body composition is not an indicator of cardiorespiratory fitness.

D) Incorrect. Muscular strength is not an indicator of cardiorespiratory fitness.

103. A) **Correct.** Income is a personal attribute.

B) Incorrect. Income is not an environmental factor.

C) Incorrect. Income cannot be considered a physical-activity factor.

D) Incorrect. Income is not a core factor.

104. A) Incorrect. The compensation of the knees would be adducted or abducted.

B) **Correct.** The compensation of the feet from the anterior view is neither flattened nor externally rotated.

C) Incorrect. The compensation of the hips is anteriorly or posteriorly rotated.

D) Incorrect. The compensation of the head is tilted or rotated.

105. A) Incorrect. The long jump test is used to measure maximal jumping distance.

B) **Correct.** The barbell squat test is used to measure lower body strength.

C) Incorrect. The overhead squat assesses dynamic flexibility.

D) Incorrect. The hexagon test is used to measure agility.

106. A) Incorrect. This is a characteristic of correct posture.

B) Incorrect. This is a characteristic of correct posture.

C) **Correct.** The shoulders should remain neutral and in line with the LPHC; the head and neck should be straight, with eyes gazing forward.

D) Incorrect. This is a characteristic of correct posture.

107. A) **Correct.** A professional trainer should wear tasteful and modest attire that is representative of the fitness industry.

B) Incorrect. A professional trainer should wear attire appropriate for the fitness industry.

C) Incorrect. The attire of a professional trainer should be tasteful and modest.

D) Incorrect. A personal trainer's attire should be clean and appear professional to clients.

108. A) **Correct.** Only 7 percent of communication is through verbal communication.

B) Incorrect. The figure of 10 percent is not accurate.

C) Incorrect. Fifty-five percent of our communication is commonly attributed to our body language.

D) Incorrect. Vocal quality makes up 38 percent of our communication.

109. A) Incorrect. This is much higher intensity than the client will ever experience while golfing.

B) Correct. Walking at varying inclines on a treadmill may mimic the layout of the golf course.

C) Incorrect. Golfers do not typically ride bicycles on the course and this is a much higher-intensity activity than is typically seen in golf.

D) Incorrect. Golfing relies on kinesthetic control; long-distance cardiovascular activity is not a factor in a golf match.

110. A) Incorrect. It is possible to use college courses to earn CEC requirements.

B) Incorrect. Industry specialization certifications can be used to obtain CEC points.

C) Correct. Contributing to a scholarly article is an acceptable way to earn CECs, but contributing to a blog is not; blogs are not considered scholarly.

D) Incorrect. It is possible to apply accredited programs' learning modules to obtain CEC points.

111. **A) Correct.** The certified fitness professional may administer the test under the guidance of the physician supervising the clinical team.

B) Incorrect. Medical treatment and procedures are the responsibility of the supervising physician.

C) Incorrect. Diagnosing symptoms is the responsibility of the supervising physician.

D) Incorrect. The certified fitness professional does not supervise the physician during testing procedures.

112. A) Incorrect. A program that focuses mainly on the upper body will not help to reduce chronic back pain.

B) Correct. Core strengthening and improving flexibility (especially in the hamstrings) can help to limit chronic back pain and should be the focus of the training program.

C) Incorrect. Lower body resistance training will not reduce lower back pain.

D) Incorrect. Avoiding the problem all together will only weaken the client and could potentially make things worse.

113. A) Incorrect. Client dissatisfaction could be related to a number of issues.

B) Incorrect. Environmental emergencies typically are unavoidable, but emergency action plans can limit liability.

C) Correct. One potential source of negligence lawsuits is equipment breakdown and the resultant injuries. This risk can be reduced with routine equipment maintenance.

D) Incorrect. Overtraining injuries are not typically due to faulty equipment.

114. A) Incorrect. Zone training eventually increases in intensity as the client progresses.

B) Incorrect. The mode can change in zone training programs.

C) Correct. It provides exercise variance through different target heart rate zones and keeps the program interesting for the client.

D) Incorrect. It does not necessarily take less time than steady state and even starts by training the client in steady state.

115. **A) Correct.** Stimulus control is a behavior modification tool to facilitate a change of habits.

B) Incorrect. Socio-ecological theory is considered a behavioral change model.

C) Incorrect. Self-monitoring does not fit the description provided.

D) Incorrect. Locus of control is not a tool to bring about behavior change.

116. A) Incorrect. The activity as described is not an example of cognitive coping.

B)   Incorrect. Self-talk is not part of social support.

C)   Correct. Using positive self-talk to acknowledge successes is an example of the relapse prevention tool.

D)   Incorrect. Time management does not include positive self-talk to acknowledge success.

117.   A)   Incorrect. The readiness-to-change model focuses on cultivating a person's self-efficacy to facilitate behavior change.

B)   Incorrect. The social cognitive theory model focuses on one person's observing a change in someone else to motivate his or her own decisions.

C)   Incorrect. While the theory of planned behavior is closely related to the description, it does not focus on the whole environment, no matter how removed, as a factor in behavior change.

D)   Correct. This is the correct descriptor for the socio-ecological model.

118.   **A)   Correct.** Accepting responsibility for one's actions is not necessarily considered a legal or ethical issue, but it is a standard that a professional trainer should maintain.

B)   Incorrect. Maintaining accurate notes on each client is an ethical standard for personal trainers.

C)   Incorrect. This is a legal or ethical standard. Personal trainers must not discriminate based on race, gender, creed, age, ability, or sexual orientation.

D)   Incorrect. Complying with sexual harassment standards is a legal or ethical standard for personal trainers.

119.   A)   Incorrect. An internal locus of control is the belief that a person has control over his or her own life.

B)   Incorrect. Intrinsic characterizes motivation.

C)   Correct. Those with an external locus of control believe that outside forces control their lives.

D)   Incorrect. This is not a locus of control descriptor.

120.   A)   Incorrect. People in the preparation phase have a moderate self-efficacy but may still feel their locus of control is external.

B)   Correct. People in the precontemplation phase have both a low self-efficacy and an external locus of control.

C)   Incorrect. People in the action phase have grown their self-efficacy to a moderate level and are shifting from an external locus of control to an internal locus of control.

D)   Incorrect. People in the termination phase have grown their self-efficacy maximally and have shifted into an internal locus of control.

121.   **A)   Correct.** The ABC model of behavior helps a person identify triggers for unwanted and desirable behaviors.

B)   Incorrect. Obsessions are not a focus of this model.

C)   Incorrect. Irritants can be considered a negative trigger, but not a positive one.

D)   Incorrect. Successes can be considered a product of using this model.

122.   A)   Incorrect. Liability insurance covers defamation.

B)   Incorrect. Liability insurance covers invasion of privacy.

C)   Incorrect. Neither liability nor miscellaneous insurance covers wrongful termination.

D)   Correct. Miscellaneous personal trainer's insurance covers bodily injury.

123.   A)   Incorrect. Kinesthetic feedback is not an actual type of feedback.

B)   Incorrect. Positive reinforcement is not necessarily specific.

C)   Correct. This is the correct description of targeted praise.

D)   Incorrect. The description is not limited to just non-verbal communication.

124. A) Incorrect. This is too much resistance.

B) Incorrect. This is too much resistance.

C) Correct. Weights during muscular power exercises should be between 0 and 60% of 1RM for safe implementation.

D) Incorrect. This is too much resistance.

125. A) Incorrect. The first transition period is between the preparatory period and competitive period.

B) Incorrect. These are not the periods; they are the cycles.

C) Incorrect. The order is incorrect.

D) Correct. The preparatory period is first, followed by the first transition period, then the competitive period, and finally the second transition period.

Go to **ascenciatestprep.com/cscs-online-resources** to take your second CSCS practice test and to access other online study resources.

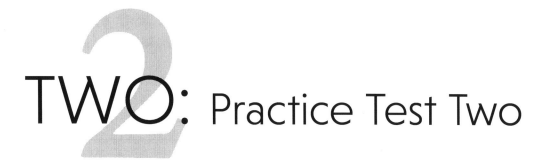

TWO: Practice Test Two

SCIENTIFIC FOUNDATIONS EXAM

READ THE QUESTION AND THEN CHOOSE THE MOST CORRECT ANSWER.

1. Which term below best describes the microscopic, self-replicating structural and functional units of an organism with many functions?

   A) cells

   B) organs

   C) tissues

   D) organisms

2. As the duration of aerobic exercise increases beyond an hour, which source(s) of energy become more important?

   A) blood glucose and blood fatty acids

   B) muscle glycogen

   C) muscle triglycerides

   D) liver and muscle glycogen

3. Proximal is the opposite of

   A) inferior.

   B) medial.

   C) dorsal.

   D) distal.

4. Which of the answer choices below does NOT describe a function of the bones?

   A) They store necessary minerals.

   B) They protect internal organs.

   C) They synthesize blood cells.

   D) They produce force for movement.

5. What is the name of the large bone found in the upper leg?

   A) femur

   B) tibia

   C) humerus

   D) fibula

6. Muscular atrophy occurs as a result of

   A) performing the same exercises every workout.

   B) lack of exercise or injury.

   C) progressively overloading the muscles with a well-developed exercise program.

   D) cardiovascular training.

7. Which term below best refers to poor bone mineral density due to the loss or lack of production of calcium content and bone cells, which leads to bone brittleness?

A) rheumatoid arthritis

B) arthritis

C) osteoporosis

D) postural deviation

8. Which answer choice below best describes the body's joints?

A) The joints are where tendons attach to muscles.

B) Joints frequently do not allow movement.

C) Joints are the long section of bones.

D) Joints are where two bones are attached by connective tissue to allow movement.

9. Waist-to-hip ratio (WHR) is an indicator of excess abdominal fat; fat carried around the waist increases the risk for obesity-related diseases more than that which is carried on the hips. A WHR greater than which of the following increases the risk of disease for men?

A) 0.86

B) 0.95

C) 0.70

D) 1.05

10. Mechanical advantage refers to

A) efficiency of a lever based on where the forces are being applied.

B) efficiency of a lever based on how much force is applied.

C) efficiency of a lever based on how far the range of motion is.

D) efficiency of a lever based on how many times a force can be applied.

11. Which *B* vitamin is central to amino acid metabolism?

A) niacin

B) pantothenic acid

C) pyridoxine

D) riboflavin

12. How much of a caloric surplus is recommended for an individual trying to gain weight as lean body mass?

A) 1,000 kcal/day

B) 700 – 800 kcal/day

C) 400 – 500 kcal/day

D) 100 – 200 kcal/day

13. Which is false? Someone who does prolonged intense exercise every day

A) will achieve maximum health.

B) may be addicted to exercise.

C) is not allowing an adequate recovery time after exercise.

D) could suffer fatigue, depression, and frequent illness.

14. Which disorder is typified by a poor body image, an overwhelming desire to lose weight despite being at a normal weight, and an extreme avoidance of food?

A) bulimia nervosa

B) exercise addiction

C) anorexia nervosa

D) fad dieting

15. Which of the following is NOT an effect of anabolic steroids?

A) enlarged breasts and shrinking testicles in men

B) a feeling of calmness

C) kidney, liver, and heart damage

D) increased facial and body hair and a deeper voice in women

16. For maximum performance, a pre-exercise meal should contain

   A) a high amount of carbohydrates, fat, and fiber.

   B) only carbohydrates.

   C) a high amount of protein, carbohydrates, and fat.

   D) a high amount of carbohydrates, a moderate amount of protein, and a low amount fat and fiber.

17. A postexercise meal containing which of the following is most effective for replenishing muscle glycogen?

   A) carbohydrates alone

   B) protein alone

   C) carbohydrates and fat

   D) carbohydrates and protein

18. Deficiency of what vitamin can lead to poor bone density?

   A) vitamin D

   B) vitamin A

   C) vitamin C

   D) vitamin K

19. Supplemental creatine might benefit a vegetarian weight lifter because

   A) it helps build muscle proteins.

   B) it is an amino acid mainly present in meat.

   C) it is plentiful in meat and improves endurance.

   D) it is plentiful in meat and can provide a burst of energy for short-duration intense exercise.

20. What causes a muscular twitch?

   A) sarcomeres

   B) the neuromuscular junction

   C) action potentials

   D) motor units

21. Performing a calf raise is an example of which type of lever?

   A) a first-class lever

   B) It is not a type of lever.

   C) a second-class lever

   D) a third-class lever

22. Carbohydrate loading is done by

   A) consuming a large quantity of carbohydrates just prior to an event.

   B) drinking sports drinks containing carbohydrates during an event.

   C) doing a fruit juice cleanse the day before an event.

   D) following a low-carbohydrate diet with the addition of exercise for three days, followed by three days of little activity with a high-carbohydrate diet.

23. Hyperextension refers to

   A) flexion beyond normal range of motion of a joint.

   B) extension through normal range of motion of a joint.

   C) rapid extension of a joint.

   D) extension beyond normal range of motion of a joint.

24. At which level does gas exchange occur?

   A) arteries

   B) veins

   C) arterioles

   D) capillaries

25. Excessive lateral curvature of the spine is referred to as

A) scoliosis.

B) lordosi.

C) osteoporosis.

D) kyphosis.

26. How many of each type of vertebrae does the spine have?

A) 9 cervical, 12 thoracic, 7 lumbar, 1 sacral

B) 12 cervical, 7 thoracic, 5 lumbar, 5 sacral

C) 5 cervical, 12 thoracic, 7 lumbar, 5 sacral

D) 7 cervical, 12 thoracic, 5 lumbar, 5 sacral

27. What happens to a person's base of support when the feet are spread apart further?

A) The base of support decreases.

B) The base of support stays the same.

C) Base of support is not related to a person's stance.

D) The base of support increases.

28. During which stage of life does bone grow more quickly?

A) childhood

B) adulthood

C) old age

D) Bone grows steadily over a lifespan.

29. What is the name of the contractile units found in muscle that are used to produce force?

A) myofibrils

B) muscle fibers

C) muscle groups

D) sarcomeres

30. Which of these is contained in the A-band?

A) actin only

B) actin and myosin

C) Z-lines

D) I-band

31. Two proprioceptors found within muscles are

A) Golgi tendon organs and muscle fibers.

B) Golgi tendon organs and muscular agonists.

C) muscle spindle fibers and muscular antagonists.

D) Golgi tendon organs and muscle spindle fibers.

32. An Olympic weightlifter who attempts a single repetition of an exercise for competition would benefit most from having which type of muscle?

A) type IIa

B) type I

C) slow-twitch

D) type IIb

33. What is the value of VO2 for 1 MET (i.e., rest/sitting quietly)?

A) 5 mL/kg body weight/min

B) 10 mL/kg body weight/min

C) 7.5 mL/kg body weight/min

D) 3.5 mL/kg body weight/min

34. The pectoralis major muscle primarily works in which plane(s) of motion?

A) transverse only

B) frontal

C) coronal

D) transverse and sagittal

35. Which two actions do the hamstring muscles perform?

A) hip extension and knee flexion

B) hip flexion and knee flexion

C) hip extension and knee extension

D) hip flexion and knee extension

36. Which of these refers to a proprioceptor found in the large area of the muscle that senses a stretch in the muscle and subsequent neuromotor response that causes a muscular contraction of the agonist muscle and a reciprocal inhibition of the antagonist muscle?

A) Golgi tendon organs

B) muscle spindle fibers

C) motor units

D) action potentials

37. Which term below describes a collection of organs with a similar function?

A) organs

B) organ systems

C) tissues

D) cells

38. Which of these refers to a muscular contraction during which the muscle resists a force as it lengthens?

A) eccentric muscle contraction

B) concentric muscle contraction

C) isotonic muscle contraction

D) isometric muscle contraction

39. Which of the following refers to muscles that assist the muscular agonists when performing a movement?

A) antagonists

B) stabilizers

C) neutralizers

D) synergists

40. An increased Q angle in females is commonly caused by

A) a small pelvis.

B) proper resistance training.

C) a large pelvis.

D) a wider base of support.

41. An example of a common force-couple found in the body is

A) the hamstrings muscle group.

B) the quadriceps of the legs and biceps of the arms.

C) the iliopsoas of the hip and the erector spinae of the vertebral column.

D) the trapezius of the neck and the rectus abdominis of the torso.

42. What type of stretching should be done prior to exercise?

A) proprioceptive neuromuscular facilitation (PNF) stretching

B) static stretching

C) ballistic stretching

D) dynamic stretching

43. The cardiovascular system is made up of

A) the heart, lungs, veins, and arteries.

B) the heart, muscles, lungs, and veins.

C) the heart, lungs, skeleton, and nerves.

D) the heart, lungs, veins, and brain.

44. Which of the following BMI ranges is considered obese?

A) 25 – 30

B) 20 – 25

C) 30 and above

D) 25 and above

45. The skeleton is

   A) made of ligaments.

   B) a collection of cartilage found in various parts of the body.

   C) the framework of structural integrity to the body's numerous biological systems.

   D) the organs that aid in the digestion of food.

46. The tricuspid valve separates

   A) the right and left ventricles.

   B) the right atrium and right ventricle.

   C) the left atrium and left ventricle.

   D) the right atrium and inferior vena cava.

47. Which of the following do red blood cells contain?

   A) platelets

   B) plasma

   C) nuclei

   D) hemoglobin

48. Which of the following blood pressure readings indicates hypotension?

   A) 120/80

   B) 140/90

   C) 90/60

   D) 110/70

49. Atherosclerosis can lead to which dangerous health conditions?

   A) postural deviations

   B) muscular imbalances

   C) heart attack and stroke

   D) obesity

50. What is the structure on a neuron that is wrapped by a myelin sheath?

   A) the dendrites

   B) the cell body

   C) the nucleus

   D) the axon

51. The Z-band determines

   A) the length of the muscle.

   B) the length of the A-band.

   C) the length of the sarcomere.

   D) the strength of the muscle.

52. Which of the following is a broad definition of many diseases that cause chronic obstruction of airflow to the lungs, including emphysema, asthma, and bronchitis?

   A) chronic obstructive pulmonary disease

   B) chronic increased blood pressure

   C) chronic obstructive pressure disease

   D) chronic obstructive platelet disease

53. Which of the following is a chronic disease involving episodic seizures due to disruption of the central nervous system?

   A) Alzheimer's disease

   B) epilepsy

   C) multiple sclerosis

   D) COPD

54. How soon after starting a resistance training program can neuromuscular benefits be seen?

   A) after the first session

   B) after several weeks

   C) after four weeks

   D) after six weeks

55. What are the chemical substances used for controlling different bodily and cellular processes released by the glands?

   A) glands

   B) neurons

   C) adrenal glands

   D) hormones

56. Which of the following does the pancreas produce and regulate the secretion of?

   A) cortisol

   B) testosterone

   C) insulin

   D) epinephrine

57. What does human growth hormone regulate?

   A) muscle and bone development

   B) calcium absorption

   C) reproductive function

   D) insulin secretion

58. Abduction and adduction typically occur in which plane of motion?

   A) transverse

   B) frontal

   C) sagittal

   D) oblique

59. Which of the following is a glucose-based energy supply that is typically synthesized and stored in the liver and skeletal muscle of the human body?

   A) blood sugar

   B) acetyl CoA

   C) creatine phosphate

   D) glycogen

60. The neuroendocrine response to exercise is elicited by

   A) working smaller muscle groups, like the biceps or triceps.

   B) performing single joint exercises, like wrist curls.

   C) performing light cardiovascular exercise, such as walking.

   D) performing large muscle group exercises, like the deadlift.

61. What are the muscular rings that help to regulate the movement of digested food through the digestive tract?

   A) the large intestine

   B) peristalsis

   C) sphincters

   D) bile

62. Where does the absorption of nutrients through digestion primarily occur?

   A) small intestine

   B) large intestine

   C) stomach

   D) mouth

63. What is the point around which movement is created in a lever system?

   A) the fulcrum

   B) the resistive force

   C) the muscular force

   D) the lever arm

64. According to the force-velocity curve, an increase in force provides improvement to

   A) muscular strength.

   B) muscular endurance.

   C) muscular power.

   D) muscular speed.

65. Center of gravity refers to
   A) the area directly under the body, including where the body contacts the ground.
   B) the area where the least amount of body weight is located.
   C) an imaginary point on the body in which body weight is completely and evenly distributed in relation to the ground.
   D) the direct center point between a person's feet.

66. What do children tend to lack when starting a training program?
   A) muscles
   B) aerobic capacity
   C) coordination
   D) need of supervision

67. What is ATP?
   A) the acid that builds up in the muscles following intense exercise bouts
   B) the energy source for all human movement
   C) the processes by which energy is created aerobically in the human body
   D) the coenzyme that enters the Krebs cycle for energy production

68. Females tend to carry more of their muscle mass in
   A) their arms.
   B) their upper body.
   C) their chest.
   D) their lower body.

69. Which muscle group elevates the scapulae?
   A) pectoralis major
   B) biceps
   C) latissimus dorsi
   D) trapezius

70. If calculated using the Harris-Benedict equation, what would the daily caloric intake be for weight maintenance for a thirty-five-year-old active female who weighs 154 lb. and is five foot eight inches tall?
   A) 2,063 kcal/day
   B) 2,091 kcal/day
   C) 1,474 kcal/day
   D) 2,294 kcal/day

71. Which of the following is NOT a macronutrient?
   A) carbohydrate
   B) protein
   C) fat
   D) vitamin

72. What might need to be taken into consideration when developing a training program for a youth sports team?
   A) difference in size of athletes
   B) difference in ages of athletes
   C) performing resistance training
   D) performing cardiovascular training

73. What signifies that a female athlete may be overtraining?
   A) the development of muscle mass
   B) exercising most days of the week
   C) the female athlete triad
   D) fatigue

74. Which of the following statements is NOT correct about proprioceptors?

A) Proprioceptors are only found in muscles.

B) They are important in muscle memory and hand-eye coordination.

C) Muscle spindles and Golgi tendon organs are two types of proprioceptors.

D) They communicate speed, angles, and balance to the central nervous system.

75. In anatomy, the term *medial* is best described as a location that is

A) toward the midline of the body.

B) away from the midline of the body.

C) toward the top of the body.

D) toward the back of the body.

76. What should be collected first by an older adult prior to starting a fitness program?

A) one-repetition maximum testing

B) a cardiovascular assessment

C) bloodwork

D) a Physical Activity Readiness Questionnaire and medical history

77. How much energy (in kcal) would an 80 kg man use if he walked briskly for one hour (at 3.3 MET) and jumped rope for five minutes (at 10.0 MET)?

A) 347 kcal

B) 825 kcal

C) 70 kcal

D) 248 kcal

78. Skeletal bones go through a remodeling process throughout the lifetime. What role do osteoclasts play in this process?

A) They form new bone.

B) They become embedded in the bone matrix.

C) They break down bone.

D) They signal to the endocrine system to release calcitonin.

79. An amino acid is

A) a nitrogen containing sugar.

B) a compound which gives some fruits their acidity.

C) a building block of proteins.

D) found in vinegar.

80. What muscular action occurs at the forearm when the palm is rotated to face upward?

A) pronation

B) supination

C) abduction

D) flexion

81. Which type of athletes might benefit from beta blockers, which are illegal in competition?

A) Olympic lifters

B) marathon runners

C) archers

D) swimmers

82. Where is the largest store of glycogen in the body?

A) skeletal muscle

B) liver

C) brain

D) heart

83. Which is the most effective and healthy way to improve body composition?

   A) a very low-calorie diet

   B) two hours of intense exercise per day

   C) behavioral changes involving healthier food choices, smaller portions, and less snacking combined with aerobic and resistance exercise three times per week

   D) walking for a half hour each day

84. What is/are the first source(s) of energy during a sprint?

   A) muscle glycogen

   B) intramuscular triglycerides

   C) phosphocreatine and ATP

   D) liver glycogen

85. How many kilocalories of energy per gram do carbohydrates and protein provide?

   A) 7 kcal/gram

   B) 9 kcal/gram

   C) 6 kcal/gram

   D) 4 kcal/gram

86. Which food group or food groups should take up half the plate according to the USDA MyPlate program?

   A) grains

   B) fruits and vegetables

   C) protein and dairy

   D) grains and fiber

87. Which term refers to the smooth inner layer of the heart?

   A) pericardium

   B) endocardium

   C) epicardium

   D) mitral valve

88. Which of the following is NOT a function of protein in the body?

   A) It makes up muscle fibers.

   B) It composes enzymes that catalyze chemical reactions.

   C) It makes up receptors in cell membranes that transmit hormonal messages to cells.

   D) It is the major structural component of cell membranes.

89. Athletes can have greater requirements for protein, vitamins, and some minerals. What is generally the best way to meet those needs?

   A) Increased activity can be supported calorically by consuming larger servings of a varied, nutrient-rich diet consisting of fruit, vegetables, whole grains, lean protein, and low-fat dairy products.

   B) Take vitamin, protein, and mineral supplements.

   C) Eat high-calorie processed foods to maintain weight.

   D) Eat lots of high-calorie snacks between meals.

90. Older adults are at a higher risk for

   A) cardiovascular incidents during exercise.

   B) DOMS after exercise.

   C) increased muscle mass from exercise.

   D) hyperextension due to increased flexibility.

91. Which of the following is NOT an electrolyte?

   A) sodium

   B) chloride

   C) calcium

   D) selenium

92. What is the formula for body mass index (BMI)?

   A) weight (lb.)^2/height (in.)

   B) weight (lb.)/height (in.)

   C) weight (kg)/height (m)^2

   D) weight (kg)/height (cm)

93. Excess abdominal fat is NOT a risk factor for which condition?

   A) type 2 diabetes

   B) osteoporosis

   C) cardiovascular disease

   D) high blood pressure

94. What is the anaerobic portion of glucose metabolism called?

   A) the TCA cycle

   B) oxidative phosphorylation

   C) beta-oxidation

   D) glycolysis

95. How much of a caloric deficit is needed to lose a pound of fat per week?

   A) 1,200 kcal/week

   B) 3,500 kcal/week

   C) 2,000 kcal/week

   D) 1,500 kcal/week

96. Anabolic steroid abuse can cause

   A) brain damage.

   B) memory loss.

   C) liver damage.

   D) muscular atrophy.

READ THE QUESTION AND THEN CHOOSE THE MOST CORRECT ANSWER.

1. What is the single-leg squat test used to assess?

   A) muscular endurance

   B) cardiorespiratory fitness

   C) single-leg functional strength

   D) bilateral lower body strength

2. The sense of where one's body is positioned in a space is called

   A) proportion.

   B) sense memory.

   C) balancing.

   D) proprioception.

3. The purpose of the star excursion balance test is to

   A) measure agility and quickness.

   B) measure maximal force production.

   C) measure upper body strength.

   D) measure dynamic balance and ankle stability.

4. In the power phase of fitness training, what is the primary training emphasis?

   A) improving muscle endurance

   B) building prime mover strength

   C) muscle speed and force production

   D) balance training

5. Which of the following exercise deterrents is NOT an environmental factor?

   A) gender

   B) time

   C) weather

   D) social support

6. The sit-and-reach test is used to measure the flexibility of which of the following muscles?

   A) shoulders and upper back

   B) shoulders and lower back

   C) quadriceps and lower back

   D) lower back and hamstrings

7. Which body fat measuring tool uses beams of different energy levels to measure bone mineral density in order to determine body fat percentage?

   A) near-infrared interactance

   B) bioelectrical impedance

   C) dual-energy x-ray absorptiometry (DEXA)

   D) skinfold calipers

8. What is voluntary commitment to an exercise program known as?

   A) exercise selection

   B) motivation

   C) exercise adherence

   D) exercise commitment

9. Which statement below does NOT describe the use of the social support behavioral modification technique?

   A) doing a positive behavior to avoid a negative consequence of a negative behavior

   B) enlist a friend to be a workout buddy

   C) create a social media group for healthy recipe swapping

   D) have a friend or a family member on-call if feeling vulnerable

10. What are the two most common anatomical sites to measure the heart rate?

    A) brachial and radial

    B) carotid and brachial

    C) radial and femoral

    D) carotid and radial

11. What should be done in addition to dynamic stretching during the warm-up process?

    A) light to moderate cardiovascular exercise

    B) plyometric exercises

    C) agility exercises

    D) resistance training

12. In general, the code of ethics for personal trainers applies to all the following areas, EXCEPT which one?

    A) professionalism

    B) confidentiality

    C) friendship

    D) business practices

13. Which of the following is NOT within a certified fitness professional's scope of practice?

    A) fitness assessment

    B) program design

    C) massage therapy

    D) goal-setting

14. The steady progression of microcycles from muscular endurance to hypertrophy, to strength, and finally to power, describes what type of periodization?

    A) undulating periodization

    B) recreational periodization

    C) linear periodization

    D) sports-specific periodization

15. Which of the following techniques is NOT used to assess body composition?

    A) body mass index (BMI)

    B) the Margaria-Kalamen test

    C) bioelectrical impedance

    D) dual-energy x-ray absorptiometry (DEXA)

16. Plyometric exercises are also referred to as

    A) strength training.

    B) force training.

    C) quickness training.

    D) power training.

17. What is an isometric movement?

    A) intensifying a certain muscle group

    B) holding a certain muscle length

    C) extending the muscle

    D) pushing a certain muscle group

18. A personal training certification typically needs to be renewed every _____ years.

    A) one

    B) four

    C) six

    D) two

19. What is the strongest predictor of exercise program adherence?

    A) goals

    B) body composition

    C) previous injury history

    D) exercise history

20. Program design for senior citizens should incorporate exercises that improve

    A) muscular power.

    B) the ability to perform daily tasks.

    C) anaerobic endurance.

    D) arm strength.

21. Fitness professionals should keep clients' emergency contact information

    A) stored in their cell phones.

    B) on an email list.

    C) filed on the work computer.

    D) alphabetized in a locked, easily accessible filing cabinet.

22. Which machines use a combination of the body's concentric and eccentric force, gravity, and the friction from the pulleys and weight loaded to dictate the speed of the machine and range of motion?

    A) free weights

    B) hydraulic machines

    C) suspension trainers

    D) cam machines

23. Which of the following is NOT a benefit of exercise testing?

    A) assessing physical work capacity

    B) assessing movement capabilities

    C) determining if a medical referral will be needed prior to exercise

    D) determining acute variables for an exercise program

24. Which of the following is NOT a potential risk factor associated with clients requiring medical clearance?

    A) sedentary lifestyle

    B) high blood pressure

    C) low resting heart rate

    D) obesity

25. The dynamic warm-up should implement exercises that

    A) prepare all of the muscles that will be trained during the workout.

    B) improve flexibility.

    C) are basic and not specific.

    D) increase muscular power.

26. Along with proper body positioning, another way to isolate muscle groups with efficiency is to use different types of _____ while lifting barbells, dumbbells, or kettlebells, and while using weight machines.

    A) weights

    B) breathing

    C) grips

    D) swings

27. A forward lunge works in what plane of motion?

    A) sagittal plane

    B) transverse plane

    C) any plane

    D) frontal plane

28. In which phases of the readiness-to-change model will clients need to use behavior modification tools to keep them on track?

    A) maintenance and termination phases

    B) action and precontemplation phases

    C) action and maintenance phases

    D) contemplation and preparation phases

29. Assisted stretching is also known as _____.

A) SMR

B) foam rolling

C) dynamic

D) PNF

30. A machine leg extension is an example of what type of movement?

A) closed kinetic chain movement

B) core exercise

C) open kinetic chain movement

D) transverse movement

31. Some personal trainers provide _____ advice, which can fall outside of their scope of practice unless they are further certified.

A) exercise

B) stretching

C) general health

D) nutrition

32. Obese clients may need to avoid which exercises due to excessive stress placed on the joints?

A) muscular power exercises, such as Olympic lifts and plyometrics

B) muscular endurance exercises with low loads and high volume

C) muscular strength exercises with heavy loads and low volumes

D) muscular hypertrophy exercises because they will increase the client's body weight, further adding to the stress

33. A static postural assessment will provide information on the following, EXCEPT

A) proper cardiovascular function.

B) joint misalignment.

C) proper muscle length.

D) possible muscular dysfunction.

34. Which exercise is most beneficial for basketball players' peak performance?

A) bench press

B) leg press

C) squat jumps

D) rotator cuff exercises

35. What is a regression for a ball crunch?

A) single-leg windmill

B) bent leg sit-up

C) abdominal crunch

D) cable rotation

36. Which of the following is NOT a movement compensation observed during the single-leg squat assessment?

A) LPHC anteriorly tilts

B) when the hip of the raised leg elevates

C) internal rotation of the standing leg's knee

D) inward rotation of the torso

37. The readiness-to-change theory differs from the other behavior change models, because it indicates _____ stages of change.

A) no

B) generalized

C) distinct

D) two

38. Overuse injuries are caused by

A) gradual progression of exercise intensity over the course of a training program.

B) rapid progression of exercise intensity or training too frequently.

C) training only once per week for thirty minutes.

D) resistance training programs focused on muscular balance.

39. Novice clients' rest periods may differ from those of advanced clients in that

A) novices will require less rest before starting the next set of an exercise.

B) novices may require more rest periods per workout than advanced clients.

C) novices should get rest periods only between different exercises but not between sets

D) novices should get rest periods only between sets but not between exercises.

40. When should PNF stretching be implemented into the program?

A) during the warm-up

B) during the resistance training phase

C) before performing cardiovascular exercise

D) during the flexibility and cooldown

41. Monitoring exercise intensity is a means of

A) making workouts more fun for clients.

B) making sure everyone is exercising at the same pace.

C) making sure the client gets good value from the training sessions.

D) reducing the risks involved with exercise.

42. The practice of active listening means _____ and _____ _____are occurring while working with a client.

A) verbal, non-verbal communication

B) positive, negative body language

C) empathy, rapport building

D) core, structural exercises

43. If a client appears to have mastered the exercise in a workout, the trainer should

A) implement a progression of the exercise the client mastered.

B) implement a regression of the exercise the client mastered.

C) stop the client from exercising.

D) implement a totally new workout.

44. What is one method for signaling and alerting emergency authorities?

A) setting off a fire alarm

B) shouting for help

C) calling a friend

D) emailing an authority figure

45. During a dynamic warm-up, the dynamic movements should include about

A) fifteen repetitions per side of each exercise.

B) one or two repetitions per side of each exercise.

C) ten to twenty repetitions per side of each exercise.

D) five repetitions per side of each exercise.

46. Which term describes using specific movements or words to inform participants of upcoming events?

A) cueing

B) exercise

C) phrasing

D) sign language

47. The pectoral is another name for what muscle?

A) chest

B) midback

C) hamstring

D) buttocks

48. What muscles are targeted in a lateral pulldown?

 A) transversus abdominis

 B) latissimus dorsi

 C) anterior deltoids

 D) quadriceps

49. Why is enjoyment important in an exercise program?

 A) It helps to improve strength.

 B) It helps to improve cardiovascular fitness.

 C) It helps with client compliance with programs.

 D) It helps to determine client goals.

50. For which type of client might the mode of cardiovascular exercise be more important?

 A) an exerciser who participates in multiple recreational activities

 B) a marathon runner

 C) an exerciser training for general health benefits

 D) an exerciser training for fitness improvement

51. What is a repetition?

 A) The performance of an exercise multiple times through its full range of motion.

 B) The amount of weight used for an exercise.

 C) The number of exercises used in a workout.

 D) The performance of an exercise through its full range of motion one time.

52. The learning stage of progression associated with the client mastering an exercise technique without movement compensations is

 A) the autonomous stage.

 B) the cognitive stage.

 C) the continual stage.

 D) the associative stage.

53. Why is it important for the personal trainer to observe movement from three angles during movement assessments?

 A) to observe gross deviations of alignment and asymmetries

 B) to observe movement in one plane of motion

 C) to understand how each client moves

 D) to determine how each individual holds his or her body during stance

54. Rest period refers to the break during workouts between which two of the following?

 A) sets and progressions

 B) sets and exercises

 C) sets and range of motion

 D) strength and endurance

55. When performing supersets, which combination of exercises would be most appropriate?

 A) lunges and step-ups

 B) push and push

 C) pull and push

 D) push-ups and bench press

56. What muscles are targeted in a cable rotation?

A) glutes

B) obliques

C) biceps brachii

D) trapezius

57. These are proper body positioning for fast feet, EXCEPT:

A) arms pumping

B) knees high

C) bodyweight on toes

D) knees locked

58. The first transition period in a training program usually occurs between

A) the preparatory period and competition period.

B) the second transition period and the preparatory period.

C) the competition period and the second preparatory period.

D) the first two microcycles.

59. The repetition range for development of muscular hypertrophy is between

A) one and five repetitions.

B) fifteen and twenty repetitions.

C) ten and fifteen repetitions.

D) eight and twelve repetitions.

60. What does *FITTE* in FITTE Principle stand for?

A) frequency, interval, time, type, enjoyment

B) fitness, interval, time, type, enjoyment

C) frequency, intensity, time, type, extracurricular

D) frequency, intensity, time, type, enjoyment

61. Which movement compensation is seen from the anterior view during the overhead squat?

A) the arms falling forward

B) an excessive forward lean

C) the lower back arching

D) the knees moving inward

62. A program containing muscular strength, muscular endurance, and muscular hypertrophy within a single microcycle is considered what?

A) linear periodization

B) undulating periodization

C) exercise regression

D) dangerous

63. An appropriate and healthy amount of weight loss for weight management clients is approximately

A) four pounds per week.

B) five pounds per week

C) unimportant.

D) about one pound per week.

64. Which two effects of cardiovascular training are consistent between aerobic and anaerobic exercise during the workout?

A) increased heart rate and lactate threshold

B) increased heart rate and type II muscle fiber recruitment

C) increased heart rate and respiration rate

D) increased blood pressure and type I muscle fiber recruitment

65. When spotting a shoulder press, where should the spotter's hands be?

A) wrists

B) elbows

C) neck

D) back

66. Assisted sprint training uses what type of implement?

A) sled

B) kettlebell

C) bungee cord

D) parachute

67. What is the most appropriate assessment for a prenatal client?

A) bench press

B) single-leg squat

C) gait

D) forty-yard dash

68. What is a regression of a kettlebell swing?

A) straight-leg deadlift

B) box jump

C) single-arm swing

D) front raise

69. An effective cooldown

A) should mimic the warm-up to ensure steady heart rate reduction.

B) should start with falling on the floor in exhaustion.

C) should still have weight training in it.

D) should have the client just walking around.

70. The technique of setting reasonable and attainable goals to inhibit unsuccessful results is an example of

A) self-monitoring.

B) cognitive coping.

C) reward.

D) negative reinforcement.

71. Improving lactate threshold can be accomplished by the trainer implementing

A) steady-state cardiovascular training.

B) maximal-strength resistance training.

C) muscular power training.

D) sprint interval training.

72. Why would riding a road bicycle not be an advisable cardiovascular training for a pregnant client?

A) It is not effective at developing cardiovascular fitness.

B) A fall could be hazardous to the unborn child and mother.

C) The intensity is too high for the client.

D) The intensity is too low for the client.

73. If the rest period is around thirty seconds and the load is light, which repetition range is most appropriate?

A) one repetition

B) eight repetitions

C) ten repetitions

D) fifteen repetitions

74. As training volume decreases, load

  A) increases.

  B) decreases.

  C) stays the same.

  D) does not change because the two variables are not associated.

75. What is the starting position for a power drop?

  A) supine

  B) sitting

  C) semi-supine

  D) prone

76. Which testing surfaces are used during the balance error scoring system?

  A) sand

  B) water

  C) balance beam

  D) foam pad

77. CEC stands for

  A) constant educational content.

  B) continuing education credit.

  C) collective exercise collaboration.

  D) care education collective.

78. What is the common PNF stretching sequence?

  A) stretch-release

  B) hold-relax

  C) relax-breathe

  D) contract-contract

79. Which of the following assessments measures muscular endurance?

  A) push-up test

  B) three-minute step test

  C) overhead squat

  D) barbell squat test

80. When using active listening, a trainer should do what after the client has finished his statement or question?

  A) Give him a high five and a smile.

  B) Give him a hug.

  C) Walk away nodding.

  D) Repeat key elements of the client's statement.

81. Where should the rules and regulations for an emergency action plan be obtained?

  A) from fitness websites

  B) from certified fitness professionals

  C) from the US Department of Labor

  D) from any local business

82. Calculations of which of the following will allow the personal trainer to target an individual's cardiorespiratory health and overall fitness level?

  A) heart rate max

  B) VO2 max

  C) body fat

  D) resting heart rate

83. What are open kinetic chain exercises?

  A) exercises that allow foot or hand movement

  B) exercises that load the spine

  C) exercises that keep either feet or hands at a fixed point

  D) exercises that rely on a partner to stretch the limbs

84. When someone initiates a plan to solve a problem within a month, that person is in the _____ phase.

  A) preparation

  B) contemplation

  C) action

  D) termination

85. Since children have difficulty regulating their body temperature, it is important to make sure

   A) they are exercising outdoors.

   B) they exercise only when it is cold out.

   C) they are hydrating properly.

   D) they are exercising indoors.

86. Which of the following tests requires a spotter?

   A) balance error scoring system

   B) single-leg squat

   C) star excursion balance test

   D) overhead squat

87. A synergist muscle _____ the prime mover during a joint action.

   A) repels

   B) connects

   C) aids

   D) forces

88. What does the *SMART* goals acronym stand for?

   A) specific, measurable, aerobic, realistic, time-stamped

   B) strength training, measurable, action-oriented, realistic, time-stamped

   C) specific, measurable, action-oriented, realistic, time-stamped

   D) specific, measurable, action-oriented, regular, time-stamped

89. Program design for athletic improvement relies heavily on

   A) exercise specificity.

   B) resistance training every day.

   C) cardiovascular training every day.

   D) the amount of weight the athlete can lift for one repetition.

90. For a training program to follow the principle of overload it needs to

   A) maintain training loads throughout the program.

   B) gradually increase training loads throughout the program.

   C) decrease training loads throughout the program.

   D) rapidly increase training loads throughout the program.

91. Injury is categorized as which type of barrier to exercise adherence?

   A) environmental factor

   B) personal attribute

   C) physical-activity factor

   D) locus of control

92. What should NOT be done during a hip sled?

   A) bending the knees

   B) raising the toes

   C) locking the knees

   D) pressing into the heels

93. Sandbags, resistance tubes, and stability balls are what types of equipment?

   A) transitional

   B) cardio

   C) functional

   D) controlled

94. What is a training plateau?

   A) a decrease in the difficulty of an exercise due to physical limitation

   B) a high point in the training program where a goal is achieved

   C) an increase in exercise difficulty designed to overload the muscles

   D) a point in a client's training program associated with no positive gains from exercise

95. Periodization programs should strive to have the athlete peak

   A) throughout the entirety of the program.

   B) at the beginning of the program.

   C) just prior to competition or major events such as tryouts.

   D) Peak performance should not be reached because it is potentially harmful to the client.

96. Which of these tests is used to measure a client's stretch-shortening cycle effort?

   A) long jump

   B) reactive strength index

   C) forty-yard dash

   D) hexagon

97. The RPE scale is a subjective scale measuring

   A) how much exercise the client is performing.

   B) what mode of exercise the client is performing.

   C) how difficult the client feels the exercise is.

   D) the client's opinion of the workout for the day.

98. An effective warm-up should last between 5 – 10 minutes at what type of intensity?

   A) moderate to high intensity

   B) multiple interval intensity

   C) low to moderate intensity

   D) high intensity

99. Which of the following is NOT a negative body language indicator?

   A) finger tapping

   B) tall posture

   C) shifting eyes

   D) arms crossed

100. Which two might be the proper regression and progression of the push-up exercise?

   A) alternating single-leg push-ups and BOSU Ball push-ups

   B) push-ups with feet elevated and clapping push-ups

   C) kneeling push-ups and wall push-ups (hands on wall)

   D) kneeling push-ups and push-ups with feet elevated

101. Placing the body under excess stress to elicit a physiological adaptation to exercise is referred to as

   A) general adaptation syndrome.

   B) specificity.

   C) overtraining.

   D) progression.

102. Regardless of whether a fitness professional is considered a gym employee, all trainers should obtain what?

   A) liability insurance

   B) a group fitness certification

   C) fitness equipment

   D) a social media account

103. During the gait assessment, which compensation could be observed at the ankle and foot checkpoints?

   A) an overpronation of the foot

   B) lifting of the heels

   C) heel strikes first

   D) stride is too short

104. Which is an alternative to standard aerobic training?

   A) plyometrics

   B) stretching

   C) core training

   D) circuit training

105. Which type of stretching helps to elicit an elongation of the muscle fibers and improved flexibility?

A) dynamic stretching

B) static stretching

C) self-myofascial release

D) dynamic warm-up

106. If a client has had a recent joint surgery, what should the trainer do before starting the fitness program?

A) a fitness assessment

B) require the client to get a physician's clearance to exercise

C) take the client through a workout and avoid the injured joint

D) tell the client to work out on his own

107. Non-verbal communication generally consists of

A) vocal tone and words.

B) body language and singing skills.

C) vocal tone and body language.

D) words and body language.

108. During the overhead squat assessment, the personal trainer observes flattening of the feet. Which of the following terms describes what the personal trainer is observing?

A) posterior pelvic tilt

B) lower crossed syndrome

C) pronation distortion syndrome

D) upper crossed syndrome

109. Basic Life Support (BLS) certification courses for fitness professionals should include training in

A) CPR only.

B) AED only.

C) first aid, CPR, and AED.

D) evaluating cardiac arrhythmias.

110. _____ and _____ can be considered the most difficult of exercise adherence barriers to overcome.

A) Income and fitness level

B) Accessibility and self-efficacy

C) Locus of control and intrinsic motivators

D) Self-efficacy and locus of control

111. In the _____ phase of change, the individual has taken definitive steps to change his or her behavior.

A) precontemplation

B) maintenance

C) action

D) preparation

112. Inconsistency of a muscle around a joint is considered a

_____.

A) muscle knot

B) muscle imbalance

C) muscle explosion

D) muscle structure

113. During an overhead squat assessment, which of the following compensations CANNOT be viewed posteriorly?

A) lateral movement of the feet

B) excessive foot pronation

C) heels lift from the floor

D) asymmetrical weight shift in the hips

114. Which of the following describes the type of validity that represents the extent to which test scores are related to those of other accepted tests that measure the same ability?

- **A)** content validity
- **B)** criterion-referenced validity
- **C)** face validity
- **D)** concurrent validity

115. Which type of muscular training should a client seeking to lose weight start with?

- **A)** muscular power
- **B)** muscular endurance
- **C)** muscular strength
- **D)** anaerobic cardiovascular training

116. Which of the following is NOT a relative contraindication?

- **A)** uncontrollable metabolic disease
- **B)** symptomatic heart failure
- **C)** musculoskeletal disorder
- **D)** history of heart illness

117. What is thoracic kyphosis?

- **A)** head forward
- **B)** back arched
- **C)** shoulders forward
- **D)** knees knocked

118. Which exercise may be more beneficial to a football player than the bench press?

- **A)** biceps curls
- **B)** seated machine shoulder press
- **C)** seated lat pull-downs
- **D)** push presses

119. Which of the following muscles is NOT part of the movement system of the core?

- **A)** transversus abdominis
- **B)** hip flexors
- **C)** erector spinae
- **D)** abductor complex

120. What types of exercises are considered dynamic stretches?

- **A)** med ball chops and prisoner squats
- **B)** barbell deadlifts and arm circles
- **C)** butt kickers and hamstring static stretch
- **D)** squat jumps and shoulder push press

121. Which exercise might be implemented in the first transition period of a triathlete's fitness program?

- **A)** alternating leg bounding plyometrics
- **B)** a standard wall sit
- **C)** barbell bench press
- **D)** tricep kickbacks

122. The RICE acronym should be followed when a person has

- **A)** injuries involving severe bleeding.
- **B)** injuries involving sprains, strains, or contusions.
- **C)** injuries involving cardiopulmonary issues.
- **D)** injuries involving chest pain.

123. How might the trainer regress a bodyweight squat exercise?

A) add weights with a vest or dumbbells

B) add a jump to the top of the range of motion

C) perform a bodyweight Romanian deadlift

D) perform a wall sit or wall slide exercise

124. Which of the following does NOT indicate a credible website for fitness articles and research?

A) .org

B) .biz

C) .edu

D) .gov

125. It is important to focus on form and _____ before loading the body with heavy weight loads.

A) body control

B) breathing

C) lengthening

D) positive outlook

1. **A)** **Correct.** This is the definition of a cell.

B) Incorrect. Organs are a collection of tissues with a similar function.

C) Incorrect. Tissues are a collection of cells with a similar function.

D) Incorrect. Organisms are a collection of organ systems that make up a living being.

2. **A)** **Correct.** As aerobic exercise progresses, muscle glycogen and triglycerides are depleted, and blood glucose and blood fatty acids account for a larger portion of energy.

B) Incorrect. Muscle glycogen is depleted as exercise progresses.

C) Incorrect. Muscle triglycerides are depleted as exercise progresses.

D) Incorrect. Glycogen stores are depleted during exercise.

3. A) Incorrect. Superior is the opposite of inferior.

B) Incorrect. Lateral is the opposite of medial.

C) Incorrect. Ventral is the opposite of dorsal.

D) **Correct.** Distal is the opposite of proximal.

4. A) Incorrect. This is a function of the bones.

B) Incorrect. This is a function of the bones.

C) Incorrect. This is a function of the bones.

D) **Correct.** Bones do NOT produce force for movement.

5. **A)** **Correct.** The large bone of the upper leg is the femur.

B) Incorrect. This bone is in the lower leg.

C) Incorrect. This bone is in the upper arm.

D) Incorrect. This bone is in the lower leg.

6. A) Incorrect. This will not induce muscular atrophy.

B) **Correct.** Lack of exercise or injury can cause muscular atrophy.

C) Incorrect. This will induce the opposite, known as muscular hypertrophy.

D) Incorrect. This will not cause muscular atrophy.

7. A) Incorrect. This is an auto-immune inflammatory attack on the joints that causes joint degeneration.

B) Incorrect. This is inflammation of the joint.

C) **Correct.** This is the definition of osteoporosis.

D) Incorrect. This is an issue with posture due to muscular imbalance.

8. A) Incorrect. This does not refer to a joint.

B) Incorrect. Most joints of the body allow for movement.

C) Incorrect. This is not a joint.

D) **Correct.** This is the definition of joints.

9. A) Incorrect. This is the value for women.

B) **Correct.** A WHR greater than 0.95 is unhealthy for men.

C) Incorrect. A WHR of 0.70 is lower than the WHR threshold for disease risk.

D) Incorrect. A WHR of 1.05 is above the WHR threshold for disease risk.

10. **A)** **Correct.** This is the definition of mechanical advantage.

B) Incorrect. This does not describe mechanical advantage.

C) Incorrect. This does not describe mechanical advantage.

D) Incorrect. This does not describe mechanical advantage.

11. A) Incorrect. Niacin is a component of the enzyme cosubstrate NAD(H), which is important in energy production.

B) Incorrect. Pantothenic acid is involved in aerobic energy metabolism, fatty acid synthesis, and the breakdown of some amino acids, but it does not play a major role in amino acid metabolism.

C) **Correct.** Pyridoxine is central to amino acid metabolism due to its involvement in transfers of amino and carboxyl groups.

D) Incorrect. Riboflavin is a component of coenzymes involved in oxidation/reduction reactions.

12. A) Incorrect. A caloric surplus of 1,000 kcal/day exceeds the body's capability to add muscle and would result in fat gain.

B) Incorrect. A caloric surplus of 700 – 800 kcal/day exceeds the body's capability to add muscle and would result in fat gain.

C) **Correct.** This is the maximum level of caloric surplus that does not exceed the body's ability to add muscle.

D) Incorrect. This amount of caloric surplus would not add significant weight.

13. A) **Correct.** Intense exercise without adequate recovery time can lead to health problems.

B) Incorrect. This is true. Some individuals believe the more they exercise—to a point of excess—the healthier they will be, and they can become addicted.

C) Incorrect. This is true. A recovery time of two days is necessary after intense exercise.

D) Incorrect. This is true. The stress of constant exercise without adequate recovery can lead to fatigue, depression, and frequent illness.

14. A) Incorrect. Bulimia nervosa involves binge eating followed by extreme compensatory behavior, like purging.

B) Incorrect. Exercise addiction involves excessive exercising, not necessarily an aversion to eating.

C) **Correct.** Anorexia nervosa involves an extreme desire for thinness and fear of weight gain with an aversion to eating.

D) Incorrect. Fad diets involve a range of inappropriate weight loss approaches, which may include starvation diets as well as abstaining from whole classes of nutrients, such as carbohydrates.

15. A) Incorrect. Enlarged breasts and shrinking testicles in men are effects of anabolic steroids.

B) **Correct.** Calmness is not an effect of anabolic steroids; they can actually cause irritability and paranoia.

C) Incorrect. Anabolic steroids can cause kidney, liver, and heart damage.

D) Incorrect. Increased facial and body hair as well as a deeper voice are effects of anabolic steroids in women.

16. A) Incorrect. Fat and fiber slow digestion and should be minimized in a pre-exercise meal.

B) Incorrect. Some protein is also beneficial.

C) Incorrect. High amounts of protein are unnecessary, and large amounts of fat should be avoided.

D) **Correct.** The meal should be high in carbohydrates to maximize glycogen storage and provide blood glucose, contain some protein, and be low in fat and fiber to ease digestion.

17. A) Incorrect. While carbohydrates are necessary, the addition of protein maximizes glycogen storage.

B) Incorrect. Carbohydrates provide glucose to make glycogen.

C) Incorrect. Fat may help replete muscle triglycerides but plays no role in glycogen production.

D) **Correct.** A combination of carbohydrates and protein results in more glycogen storage than either does alone. Some fat may also be beneficial to replete muscle triglycerides.

18. A) **Correct.** Vitamin D regulates calcium and phosphate absorption in the intestine as well as their excretion by

the kidneys; it also regulates mineral deposition and mobilization from bone.

B) Incorrect. Vitamin A deficiency does not manifest itself in bone effects.

C) Incorrect. Vitamin C deficiency can cause bone weakness due to decreased collagen in the bone, but it does not decrease bone mineralization.

D) Incorrect. Vitamin K is involved in bone formation, but problems in blood clotting show up well before bone problems caused by deficiency, which are rare.

19. A) Incorrect. Creatine does not help build muscle protein.

B) Incorrect. Creatine is not an amino acid.

C) Incorrect. Creatine has no role in fueling exercise beyond the first brief period.

D) Correct. The main source of creatine is meat. It is used in muscle to produce creatine phosphate, which is a phosphate reservoir that can be used to produce the energy molecule ATP from ADP during the initial burst of exertion.

20. A) Incorrect. The sarcomeres do not cause a muscular twitch but contract when one occurs.

B) Incorrect. This part of the motor unit is involved in a muscular twitch but does not cause them.

C) Correct. Action potentials are the stimuli that create a muscular twitch.

D) Incorrect. The muscular twitch occurs throughout the entirety of the motor unit, but the action potential is the stimulus to create the twitch.

21. A) Incorrect. This is not an example of a first-class lever.

B) Incorrect. The calf raise utilizes a type of lever.

C) Correct. The calf raise is an example of a second-class lever.

D) Incorrect. This is not an example of a third-class lever.

22. A) Incorrect. Carbohydrate loading is a strategy used over several days prior to an event.

B) Incorrect. This is normal hydration and fuel supply during an event, not carbohydrate loading.

C) Incorrect. Cleansing has nothing to do with carbohydrate loading.

D) Correct. This procedure is designed to deplete muscle glycogen and then drive repletion to the maximum possible level.

23. A) Incorrect. Hyperextension is not flexion.

B) Incorrect. This refers to extension but not hyperextension.

C) Incorrect. The rate does not necessarily make a difference in hyperextension.

D) Correct. Hyperextension is extension beyond normal range of motion.

24. AA) Incorrect. Gas exchange does not occur here.

B) Incorrect. Gas exchange does not occur here.

C) Incorrect. Gas exchange does not occur here.

D) Correct. Gas exchange occurs in the capillaries.

25. **A) Correct.** This is the definition of scoliosis.

B) Incorrect. This is excessive anterior curvature of the spine.

C) Incorrect. This is decreased bone mineral density leading to bone brittleness.

D) Incorrect. This is excessive posterior curvature of the spine.

26. A) Incorrect. This answer choice has too many cervical and lumbar vertebrae and too few sacral vertebrae.

B) Incorrect. This answer choice has too many cervical vertebrae and too few thoracic vertebrae.

C) Incorrect. This answer choice has too few cervical vertebrae and too many lumbar vertebrae.

D) **Correct.** These are the correct number of vertebrae per section.

27. A) Incorrect. The base of support decreases when the feet are closer together.

B) Incorrect. Stance width changes the base of support.

C) Incorrect. The base of support is directly related to stance.

D) **Correct.** The base of support increases with a wider foot stance.

28. A) **Correct.** Bone grows more quickly during childhood.

B) Incorrect. Bone grows more quickly during childhood than adulthood.

C) Incorrect. Bone begins to become frailer with old age.

D) Incorrect. Bone can be maintained more easily with exercise over a lifespan, but it grows fastest during childhood.

29. A) Incorrect. Myofibrils contain the contractile units.

B) Incorrect. Muscle fibers contain the myofibrils.

C) Incorrect. The term *muscle groups* describes many muscles working together to perform an action, rather than the individual units.

D) **Correct.** Sarcomeres are the individual contractile units found in myofibrils.

30. A) Incorrect. The A-band contains myosin as well.

B) **Correct.** The A-band contains both actin and myosin.

C) Incorrect. These separate sarcomeres, and the A-band does contain Z-lines.

D) Incorrect. The I-band does not contain actin and is separate from the A-band.

31. A) Incorrect. Muscle fibers is incorrect.

B) Incorrect. Muscular agonists is incorrect.

C) Incorrect. Muscular antagonists is incorrect.

D) **Correct.** These two are muscular proprioceptors.

32. A) Incorrect. Type IIb muscles are more beneficial.

B) Incorrect. Type I muscle would not provide much benefit.

C) Incorrect. Slow-twitch fibers are the same as type I and won't benefit the lifter much.

D) **Correct.** Olympic weightlifters benefit most from having type IIb muscle fibers for maximal power output.

33. A) Incorrect. The correct value is 3.5 mL/ kg body weight/min.

B) Incorrect. The correct value is 3.5 mL/ kg body weight/min.

C) Incorrect. The correct value is 3.5 mL/ kg body weight/min.

D) **Correct.** The VO2 of 3.5 mL/ kg body weight/min is the oxygen usage defined as 1 MET (metabolic equivalent) and is equal to the value achieved when rest/sitting quietly.

34. A) Incorrect. The pectoralis major works in multiple planes, including the transverse and sagittal.

B) Incorrect. The pectoralis major does not primarily work in the frontal plane.

C) Incorrect. The frontal and coronal planes are the same, and the pectoralis major muscle does not primarily work in them.

D) **Correct.** The pectoralis major muscle primarily works in the transverse and sagittal planes.

35. A) **Correct.** These are the two primary actions of the hamstring muscles.

B) Incorrect. Hip flexion is incorrect.

C) Incorrect. Knee extension is incorrect.

D) Incorrect. Both hip flexion and knee extension are incorrect.

36. A) Incorrect. This is a proprioceptor, but not the correct proprioceptor.

B) **Correct.** This is the definition of muscle spindle fibers.

C) Incorrect. This is not a proprioceptor.

D) Incorrect. This is not a proprioceptor.

37. A) Incorrect. This is a collection of tissues with a similar function.

B) **Correct.** This is the definition of an organ system.

C) Incorrect. This is a collection of cells with a similar function.

D) Incorrect. This is the small, self-replicating unit of structure and function of the body.

38. **A)** **Correct.** This is the definition of eccentric muscle contraction.

B) Incorrect. This is the wrong type of muscle contraction.

C) Incorrect. This is the wrong type of muscle contraction.

D) Incorrect. This is the wrong type of muscle contraction.

39. A) Incorrect. These do not assist the agonists.

B) Incorrect. These prevent unwanted compensatory movement rather than assist in primary movement.

C) Incorrect. These muscles help stabilize joints during exercises.

D) **Correct.** This is the definition of synergists.

40. A) Incorrect. This generally causes a smaller Q angle.

B) Incorrect. Proper resistance training can help with an increased Q angle.

C) **Correct.** A larger pelvis can increase Q angle in females.

D) Incorrect. This is not a common cause of increased Q angle in females.

41. A) Incorrect. This is a single muscle group.

B) Incorrect. The two muscle groups do not work as a force couple to perform the same action at a joint.

C) **Correct.** These two muscles both create an anterior pelvic tilt when they contract together.

D) Incorrect. The two muscle groups do not work as a force couple to perform the same action at a joint.

42. A) Incorrect. This type of stretching was not discussed and should not be done prior to exercise.

B) Incorrect. Static stretching can limit performance and should be done after exercise.

C) Incorrect. This type of stretching was not discussed and should not be done prior to exercise.

D) **Correct.** Dynamic stretching should be done prior to exercise to improve muscle elasticity.

43. **A)** **Correct.** The cardiovascular system contains these four components.

B) Incorrect. Muscles is incorrect.

C) Incorrect. Skeleton and nerves are incorrect.

D) Incorrect. Brain is incorrect.

44. A) Incorrect. The overweight range is 25 – 29.9.

B) Incorrect. A BMI between 18.5 – 24.9 is considered healthy.

C) **Correct.** A BMI of thirty or over indicates obesity.

D) Incorrect. This includes both the overweight and obesity range.

45. A) Incorrect. The skeleton contains ligaments but is not only ligaments.

B) Incorrect. This refers to the dense connective tissue that helps support and cushion bones.

C) **Correct.** This is the definition of the skeleton.

D) Incorrect. This refers to the digestive system.

46. A) Incorrect. This valve does not separate ventricles.

B) **Correct.** The tricuspid valve separates the right atrium and right ventricle.

C) Incorrect. This is the mitral valve.

D) Incorrect. This valve does not separate the vena cava and heart.

47. A) Incorrect. Platelets are found in the bloodstream, not the red blood cells.

B) Incorrect. Plasma is found in the bloodstream, not the red blood cells.

C) Incorrect. Red blood cells are enucleated.

D) Correct. Red blood cells contain hemoglobin for oxygen transport.

48. A) Incorrect. This is healthy blood pressure.

B) Incorrect. This is hypertension.

C) Correct. This blood pressure indicates hypotension.

D) Incorrect. This is still within a healthy range of blood pressure.

49. A) Incorrect. Postural deviations are caused by atherosclerosis.

B) Incorrect. Muscular imbalances are not caused by atherosclerosis.

C) Correct. Atherosclerosis can lead to a heart attack or stroke.

D) Incorrect. Obesity is not caused by atherosclerosis.

50. A) Incorrect. The dendrites do not have myelin sheaths.

B) Incorrect. The cell body does not have a myelin sheath.

C) Incorrect. The nucleus does not have a myelin sheath.

D) Correct. The axon is covered in a myelin sheath.

51. A) Incorrect. The length of the muscle is not determined by the Z-band.

B) Incorrect. The length of the Z-band does not determine the length of the A-band.

C) Correct. The Z-bands separate sarcomeres and determine the distance between sarcomeres.

D) Incorrect. The Z-bands do not control the strength of the muscle.

52. **A) Correct.** This is the definition of chronic obstructive pulmonary disease.

B) Incorrect. Chronic increased blood pressure is incorrect.

C) Incorrect. The word pressure is incorrect.

D) Incorrect. The word platelet is incorrect.

53. A) Incorrect. This disease involves memory loss and dementia.

B) Correct. Epilepsy involves episodic seizures and disruption of the central nervous system.

C) Incorrect. This involves the breakdown of myelin sheaths of axons.

D) Incorrect. This is a chronic obstructive disorder affecting the airways of the respiratory system.

54. A) Incorrect. This is too soon.

B) Correct. After several weeks of resistance training, neuromuscular coordination is improved.

C) Incorrect. The benefits can been seen sooner than four weeks.

D) Incorrect. The benefits can be seen sooner than six weeks.

55. A) Incorrect. The glands secrete this chemical substance.

B) Incorrect. Neurons are a part of the nervous system.

C) Incorrect. The adrenal glands secrete chemical substances that control these functions.

D) Correct. This is the definition of a hormone.

56. A) Incorrect. This hormone is produced by the adrenal glands.

B) Incorrect. This hormone is produced by the testes.

C) Correct. This hormone is produced and secreted by the pancreas.

D) Incorrect. This hormone is produced by the adrenal glands.

57. **A)** **Correct.** Human growth hormone regulates muscle and bone development.

    B) Incorrect. This is regulated by parathyroid hormones.

    C) Incorrect. This is not the function of human growth hormone.

    D) Incorrect. This is regulated by the pancreas.

58. A) Incorrect. They do not typically occur in this plane of motion.

    B) **Correct.** Abduction and adduction typically occur in the frontal plane.

    C) Incorrect. They do not typically occur in this plane of motion.

    D) Incorrect. They do not typically occur in this plane of motion.

59. A) Incorrect. This is glucose.

    B) Incorrect. This is the coenzyme that goes through the Krebs cycle.

    C) Incorrect. This is used for immediate synthesis of ATP in the muscles within the first seconds of exercise.

    D) **Correct.** This is the definition of glycogen.

60. A) Incorrect. This will not likely elicit the neuroendocrine response to exercise.

    B) Incorrect. This will not likely elicit the neuroendocrine response to exercise.

    C) Incorrect. This is not an intense enough activity to elicit the neuroendocrine response to exercise.

    D) **Correct.** Large muscle group, high-intensity exercise will elicit the neuroendocrine response to exercise.

61. A) Incorrect. The tube-like large intestine is not a sphincter.

    B) Incorrect. This is the process by which food is moved through the digestive tract.

    C) **Correct.** This is the definition of a sphincter.

    D) Incorrect. This is the fluid secreted by the gallbladder that buffers stomach acid.

62. **A)** **Correct.** The small intestine is where most nutrient absorption occurs.

    B) Incorrect. The large intestine is where most water absorption occurs.

    C) Incorrect. Very little is absorbed through the walls of the stomach.

    D) Incorrect. The mouth is the site of food mastication, but little absorption occurs here.

63. **A)** **Correct.** The fulcrum is the point around which movement is created in a lever system.

    B) Incorrect. This is the weight that is being applied to the lever arm.

    C) Incorrect. This is the force being applied to the lever arm.

    D) Incorrect. This is the arm on which the forces are applied that is attached to the fulcrum.

64. **A)** **Correct.** The higher the force applied, the more emphasis on muscular strength.

    B) Incorrect. Muscular endurance is not relevant to the force-velocity curve.

    C) Incorrect. Muscular power relies on a combination of force and velocity.

    D) Incorrect. Muscular speed relies heavily on velocity of movement.

65. A) Incorrect. This refers to base of support.

    B) Incorrect. This does not accurately describe center of gravity.

    C) **Correct.** This is the definition of center of gravity.

    D) Incorrect. This is not an accurate representation of center of gravity.

66. A) Incorrect. All human beings have muscles.

    B) Incorrect. Aerobic capacity is not typically an issue in children.

    C) **Correct.** Children tend to lack the same coordination as adults.

    D) Incorrect. Children should always be supervised during training sessions.

67. A) Incorrect. This refers to lactic acid.

B) **Correct.** This is the energy source created by the body for human movement.

C) Incorrect. This refers to the Krebs cycle and electron transport chain.

D) Incorrect. This refers to acetyl CoA.

68. A) Incorrect. This is more common in males.

B) Incorrect. This is more common in males.

C) Incorrect. This is more common in males.

D) **Correct.** Females tend to carry more of their muscle mass in their lower body.

69. A) Incorrect. The pectoralis major does not elevate the scapulae.

B) Incorrect. The biceps do not elevate the scapulae.

C) Incorrect. The latissimus dorsi do not elevate the scapulae.

D) **Correct.** The trapezius muscles elevate and upwardly rotate the scapula.

70. **A)** **Correct.** $655 + 9.6 \times 70$ kg $+ 1.8 \times 173$ cm $- 4.7 \times 35$ years $= 1,474$ kcal/day

$1,474$ kcal/day $\times 1.4$ (multiplier for active individuals) $= 2,063$ kcal/day

B) Incorrect. This figure was reached because pounds were not converted to kilograms, and inches were not converted to centimeters.

C) Incorrect. This figure was reached because 1.4 was not used as the multiplier for activity.

D) Incorrect. This figure is incorrect because the equation used leaves out the age term.

71. A) Incorrect. Carbohydrates are consumed in relatively large quantities—hundreds of grams per day—to fuel metabolism and exercise, which makes them macronutrients.

B) Incorrect. Protein is a macronutrient and is required in the tens to over a hundred grams per day to maintain body structure and function.

C) Incorrect. Fat typically is consumed in tens of grams per day—about 30 percent of caloric intake—and is a major structural component of the body, comprising cell membranes and cushioning the organs. It is a macronutrient.

D) **Correct.** Vitamins are micronutrients; they are only required in small quantities, typically micrograms to milligrams per day.

72. A) Incorrect. Sizes of athletes will vary, but that does not necessarily mean they cannot perform the same exercises.

B) **Correct.** The age of the athletes will make a difference in their development, and older athletes may start to develop coordination before the younger athletes on a sports team.

C) Incorrect. As long as they are cleared for exercise by a physician, resistance training is safe for youths.

D) Incorrect. As long as they are cleared for exercise by a physician, cardiovascular training is safe for youths.

73. A) Incorrect. Development of muscle mass is a normal sign of training.

B) Incorrect. Exercising most days of the week can be safe if done properly.

C) **Correct.** The female athlete triad is a sign that a female athlete may be overtraining.

D) Incorrect. Fatigue occurs as a result of training; however, excessive fatigue may be harmful.

74. **A)** **Correct.** Proprioceptors can be found in the inner ear, synovial joints, skeletal framework, tendons, and muscle.

B) Incorrect. Development of muscle memory and hand-eye coordination are related to proprioceptors.

C) Incorrect. Muscle spindles sense muscle stretching and Golgi tendon organs sense muscle tension.

D) Incorrect. Because of communication to the CNS, movements are coordinated.

75. **A)** **Correct.** The term *medial* means toward the midline of the body.

B) Incorrect. This refers to lateral.

C) Incorrect. This refers to superior.

D) Incorrect. This refers to posterior.

76. A) Incorrect. This may not be safe for an older adult prior to starting a fitness program.

B) Incorrect. This may not be safe for an older adult prior to starting a fitness program.

C) Incorrect. This is out of the scope of a fitness professional.

D) **Correct.** These documents will help the fitness professional to assess whether the individual is healthy enough to start a fitness program or if the person requires medical clearance from a physician.

77. **A)** **Correct.** For every liter of oxygen consumed, 5 kcal are burned. [(3.3 × 3.5 mL/kg/min × 80 kg × 60 min) + (10.0 × 3.5 mL/kg/min × 80 kg × 5 min)]× 1 L/1000 mL × 5 kcal/1 L oxygen = 347 kcal

B) Incorrect. This is more energy than would be used.

C) Incorrect. This energy expenditure is far too low.

D) Incorrect. This is close to the value just for the walking.

78. A) Incorrect. Osteoblasts form new bone.

B) Incorrect. Osteoblasts get embedded in bone matrix and then become identified as osteocytes.

C) **Correct.** Osteoclasts break down bone for remodeling.

D) Incorrect. It is calcitonin that signals to the osteoclasts to begin breaking down bone.

79. A) Incorrect. An amino acid is a carboxylic acid with an amino group on the carbon next to the acid group.

B) Incorrect. Citric acid is a compound which gives some fruits their acidity.

C) **Correct.** Amino acids are joined together by peptide bonds to produce proteins.

D) Incorrect. Acetic acid is found in vinegar.

80. A) Incorrect. This is when the palm is rotated toward the ground.

B) **Correct.** This is the definition of supination.

C) Incorrect. This occurs when a limb is pulled away from the midline of the body.

D) Incorrect. This occurs as a joint angle is decreased through muscle contraction.

81. A) Incorrect. Beta blockers slow the heart and would put Olympic lifters at a disadvantage.

B) Incorrect. Because beta blockers slow the heart, they would impair running performance.

C) **Correct.** Beta blockers slow the heart, so they would be a disadvantage for athletes who exert themselves heavily. They have a calming effect that may be desirable to athletes who need steady hands, like archers, shooters, and golfers.

D) Incorrect. Swimming demands optimum cardiac output. Beta blockers would be a disadvantage.

82. **A)** **Correct.** Skeletal muscle has the largest reservoir of glycogen in the body.

B) Incorrect. The liver is the second most significant site of glycogen storage in the body.

C) Incorrect. The brain stores relatively small amounts of glycogen.

D) Incorrect. The heart does not have significant glycogen stores.

83. A) Incorrect. A very low-calorie diet is not sustainable in the long term and may not provide adequate nutrients.

B) Incorrect. This amount of exercise may not be sustainable. The body also needs a day or two to recover from intense exercise.

C) **Correct.** A combination of a moderate dietary caloric deficit achieved with smaller amounts of nutrient-rich foods, combined with weight-bearing aerobic exercise (and possibly also resistance exercise) is the best way to lose fat and increase lean body mass.

D) Incorrect. While this would be a good step for a sedentary individual and could be expected to have some health benefits, it would not create enough of a caloric deficit alone to significantly affect weight.

84. A) Incorrect. Muscle glycogen becomes important at middle distances.

B) Incorrect. Intramuscular triglycerides become important at middle distances.

C) **Correct.** These are the most readily available sources of energy and are first used in a sprint.

D) Incorrect. Liver glycogen becomes important at long distances where muscle glycogen and blood glucose are depleted.

85. A) Incorrect. This is the energy for alcohol.

B) Incorrect. This is the energy for fat.

C) Incorrect. Carbohydrates and protein both provide 4 kcal/gram.

D) **Correct.** Carbohydrates and protein both provide 4 kcal/gram.

86. A) Incorrect. While grains were the largest component of overall diet in the Food Guide Pyramid, they only occupy about a quarter of the plate in the more recent MyPlate program.

B) **Correct.** The MyPlate program places an emphasis on consuming fruits and vegetables.

C) Incorrect. Protein takes up a bit less than a quarter of the plate, and dairy is represented as a small portion to the side of the plate.

D) Incorrect. Fiber is not a food group but is present in fruit, vegetables, and grains.

87. A) Incorrect. This is the outer layer of the heart.

B) **Correct.** The endocardium is the smooth inner layer of the heart.

C) Incorrect. This is the middle layer of the heart.

D) Incorrect. This is a valve that prevents the backflow of blood from the left atrium to the left ventricle.

88. A) Incorrect. Contractile proteins are major components of muscle fibers.

B) Incorrect. Enzymes are special types of proteins that catalyze reactions.

C) Incorrect. Many membrane receptors are proteins.

D) **Correct.** Cell membranes are composed primarily of phospholipids, not protein.

89. A) **Correct.** A balanced, nutrient-rich diet that supplies adequate calories will meet most nutritional needs. Sport drinks containing electrolytes may be useful when electrolytes and fluids are lost through sweating.

B) Incorrect. Supplements are usually not necessary with a healthy diet. They may be useful if the individual is undereating, but caution needs to be taken to avoid excessive amounts of the vitamins, proteins, or minerals contained in the supplements.

C) Incorrect. Processed, refined foods lack many of the beneficial nutrients that whole foods provide.

D) Incorrect. Snacking can be healthy if nutrient-rich foods are chosen, but foods high in calories and low in fiber, vitamins, and minerals should be avoided.

90. A) **Correct.** Older adults are at a higher risk of cardiovascular incidents during exercise.

B) Incorrect. DOMS occurs at all ages.

C) Incorrect. This is a benefit of exercise rather than a risk.

D) Incorrect. Flexibility more often decreases with age due to inactivity and the need for rest.

91. A)   Incorrect. Sodium ions circulate in the blood as electrolytes.

    B)   Incorrect. Chloride ions circulate in the blood as electrolytes.

    C)   Incorrect. Calcium ions circulate in the blood as electrolytes.

    D)   Correct. Electrolytes are charged minerals that circulate in the blood. Sodium, chloride, and calcium all circulate in this form. Selenium is a component of enzymes and proteins and does not circulate in ionized form.

92. A)   Incorrect. BMI is calculated in metric units and height is squared, not weight.

    B)   Incorrect. BMI is calculated in metric units and height is squared.

    C)   Correct. BMI equals weight in kilograms divided by height squared in meters.

    D)   Incorrect. Height is squared and measured in meters, not centimeters.

93. A)   Incorrect. Excess abdominal fat is a risk factor for type 2 diabetes.

    B)   Correct. Excess abdominal fat increases the risk for type 2 diabetes, cardiovascular disease, and high blood pressure. Excess weight on the other hand increases the load on the bones and can have a stimulating effect on bone mass.

    C)   Incorrect. Excess abdominal fat is a risk factor for cardiovascular disease.

    D)   Incorrect. Excess abdominal fat is a risk factor for high blood pressure.

94. A)   Incorrect. The TCA cycle follows glycolysis and is aerobic, meaning it requires oxygen.

    B)   Incorrect. Oxidative phosphorylation is the final process in aerobic metabolism, during which oxygen serves as the final electron acceptor and reacts to form water.

    C)   Incorrect. Beta-oxidation is the aerobic pathway of fat metabolism.

    D)   Correct. Glycolysis is the first part of glucose metabolism and derives energy without requiring oxygen.

95. A)   Incorrect. A 1,200 kcal deficit will only result in the loss of about a third of a pound.

    B)   Correct. A pound of fat contains about 3,500 kcal. A caloric deficit of at least 3,500 kcal is therefore necessary to lose one pound.

    C)   Incorrect. A 2,000 kcal deficit is not enough to cause loss of a pound.

    D)   Incorrect. A 1,500 kcal deficit will result in loss of almost half a pound.

96. A)   Incorrect. This is not a common side effect of anabolic steroid abuse.

    B)   Incorrect. This is not a common side effect of anabolic steroid abuse.

    C)   Correct. Anabolic steroid abuse can damage the liver.

    D)   Incorrect. This is not a common side effect of anabolic steroid abuse.

PRACTICE TEST TWO PRACTICAL/APPLIED ANSWER KEY

1.
A) Incorrect. The repetitions of the test are not enough to assess muscular endurance.

B) Incorrect. The single-leg squat does not assess cardiorespiratory fitness.

C) Correct. One of the components the single-leg squat test measures is single-leg strength.

D) Incorrect. The single-leg squat test measures unilateral leg strength.

2.
A) Incorrect. Proportion is a part, share, or number considered in comparative relation to a whole.

B) Incorrect. Sense memory is a psychological term.

C) Incorrect. Balancing is how an individual would measure his or her proprioception.

D) Correct. Proprioception is the ability to sense where one's body is positioned in a space.

3.
A) Incorrect. The *t*-test does this.

B) Incorrect. The reactive strength index test does this.

C) Incorrect. The bench press assessment does this.

D) Correct. The star excursion balance test measures dynamic balance and ankle stability.

4.
A) Incorrect. Stabilization and strength training, not power training, focus on improving muscle endurance.

B) Incorrect. Strength training, not power training, focuses on building prime mover strength.

C) Correct. Power training focuses on muscle speed and force production.

D) Incorrect. Stabilization training, not power training, focuses on balance training.

5.
A) Correct. Gender is a personal attribute and not an environmental factor.

B) Incorrect. Time is an environmental factor.

C) Incorrect. Weather is also an environmental factor that can be an exercise deterrent.

D) Incorrect. Social support is considered an environmental factor.

6.
A) Incorrect. The shoulders and upper back are not muscles that are assessed during the sit-and-reach test.

B) Incorrect. The shoulders are not assessed, but lower back flexibility is measured.

C) Incorrect. The quadriceps are not assessed, but lower back flexibility is measured.

D) Correct. Lower back and hamstring flexibility is assessed during the sit-and-reach test.

7.
A) Incorrect. Near-infrared interactance uses probes that are placed against the body that emit light that passes through muscle and fat.

B) Incorrect. Bioelectrical impedance uses a low-level signal from electrodes that measure the electrical signal that passes through water that is present in muscle tissue.

C) Correct. The DEXA scan uses two x-ray beams of different energy levels to measure bone density.

D) Incorrect. Skinfold calipers are used to manually determine body fat percentage.

8.
A) Incorrect. *Exercise selection* is not a real term.

B) Incorrect. This is not the correct description of motivation.

C) Correct. Exercise adherence involves a voluntary commitment to an exercise program.

D) Incorrect. Exercise commitment is not an actual term, just a rewording of the description.

9. **A)** **Correct.** This describes negative reinforcement.

B) Incorrect. Finding a workout buddy is a demonstration of the social support technique.

C) Incorrect. Creating a social media group would be considered a social support technique.

D) Incorrect. Asking a friend or family member for support is one method in the social support technique.

10. **A)** Incorrect. The radial pulse point is commonly used but not the brachial pulse point.

B) Incorrect. The carotid pulse point is commonly used but not the brachial pulse point.

C) Incorrect. The radial pulse point is commonly used but not the femoral pulse point.

D) **Correct.** The carotid and radial pulse are the two most commonly used pulse points.

11. **A)** **Correct.** Light to moderate cardiovascular exercise provides blood flow to the large muscle groups, making them more elastic and pliable for exercise.

B) Incorrect. Plyometrics are high intensity and could cause injury prior to dynamic stretching.

C) Incorrect. Agility exercises are high intensity and could cause injury prior to dynamic stretching.

D) Incorrect. Resistance training should be done after the warm-up and higher intensity exercises, such as plyometrics and agility training.

12. **A)** Incorrect. Standards of professionalism are included in the code of ethics for personal trainers.

B) Incorrect. The code of ethics for personal trainers includes standards for confidentiality.

C) **Correct.** Standards for friendship are not included in the code of ethics for personal trainers.

D) Incorrect. The code of ethics for personal trainers includes standards for business practices.

13. A) Incorrect. Fitness assessment is within a personal trainer's scope of practice.

B) Incorrect. Program design is within a personal trainer's scope of practice.

C) **Correct.** Massage therapy is not within a personal trainer's scope of practice

D) Incorrect. Goal-setting is within a personal trainer's scope of practice.

14. A) Incorrect. Undulating periodization involves varying training protocols within a microcycle rather than for full microcycles.

B) Incorrect. This does not describe a type of periodization.

C) **Correct.** Steady progression of microcycles from endurance to power is a linear periodization.

D) Incorrect. Linear periodizations can be used for non-athlete clients.

15. A) Incorrect. Body mass index measurements are used to assess body composition.

B) **Correct.** The Margaria-Kalamen test is used to assess muscular power.

C) Incorrect. Bioelectrical impedance is a method used to assess body composition.

D) Incorrect. The DEXA scan is used assess body composition.

16. A) Incorrect. Strength training is also known as resistance training.

B) Incorrect. Force training is not a type of training.

C) Incorrect. Quickness training is also known as reactive training.

D) **Correct.** Plyometrics is sometimes referred to as power training because it uses explosive movements.

17. A) Incorrect. This does not describe a muscle movement.

B) **Correct.** Isometric movement means to hold the muscle at a certain length.

C) Incorrect. Extending the muscle is eccentric movement.

D) Incorrect. Pushing a certain muscle group is fatiguing it.

18. A) Incorrect. One year is not the correct renewal requirement.

B) Incorrect. Four years is not the correct renewal requirement for a personal training certification.

C) Incorrect. Six years is not correct.

D) **Correct.** A personal training certification needs to be renewed every two years.

19. A) Incorrect. Client goals will not predict exercise program adherence.

B) Incorrect. Body composition is not a predictor of exercise program adherence.

C) Incorrect. Previous injury history could be a predictor of exercise program adherence but is not the strongest.

D) **Correct.** Exercise history is the strongest predictor of exercise program adherence since it will detail previous exercise habits.

20. A) Incorrect. Muscular power exercises may be too high intensity or high impact for senior citizens.

B) **Correct.** Exercises that make the activities of daily living easier are most beneficial for senior citizens and can help prevent injuries and falls.

C) Incorrect. Anaerobic endurance training may be too high intensity for senior citizens and may not be necessary to implement in their exercise program.

D) Incorrect. Arm strength may benefit seniors in some way, but due to difficulties with balance, a total body routine is more beneficial.

21. A) Incorrect. Information stored on a trainer's phone is not accessible to other employees and could be lost if the phone is damaged.

B) Incorrect. Keeping the information on an email list does not allow for quick access to the information in emergency situations.

C) Incorrect. Work computers often have multiple users, and the emergency contact information could be lost among the files or accessed by another user, compromising client privacy.

D) **Correct.** Keeping files alphabetized in a filing cabinet allows for easy access in case of an emergency, and locking the cabinet ensures the files stay secure.

22. A) Incorrect. Free weights use gravity and the body's concentric and isometric force.

B) Incorrect. Hydraulic machines use compressed air or water resistance.

C) Incorrect. Suspension trainers use bodyweight, gravity, and leverage.

D) **Correct.** Cam machines use a combination of body movement, gravity, and friction to work the body.

23. A) Incorrect. Exercise testing will measure physical work capacity.

B) Incorrect. Exercise testing will assess movement capabilities.

C) **Correct.** The initial interview will determine if a medical referral is needed, not exercise testing.

D) Incorrect. Exercise testing will help the personal trainer select the proper acute variables for the client's exercise program.

24. A) Incorrect. A sedentary lifestyle is a potential risk factor.

B) Incorrect. High blood pressure is a risk factor that may require the client to get medical clearance.

C) **Correct.** A low resting heart rate is NOT a risk factor that could require medical clearance.

D) Incorrect. Obesity is a risk factor, and new clients with this condition may require medical clearance.

25. **A)** **Correct.** The dynamic warm-up should be specific to the exercise performed in the workout.

B) Incorrect. Flexibility is improved by static stretching, which should be performed after the workout.

C) Incorrect. Specific movement preparation will better prepare the body for specific movements. A basic general warm-up may not adequately prepare the body for the excess stress of the workout and may lead to injury or poor performance.

D) Incorrect. Exercises for muscular power should be performed during the workout, not the warm-up.

26. A) Incorrect. Weight loads do not have any bearing on muscle isolation.

B) Incorrect. While breathing is a component of exercise technique, it is unrelated to muscle isolation.

C) **Correct.** The way the athlete grips barbells, machines, or free weights can help isolate muscle groups.

D) Incorrect. This is a way to use free weights, and can be combined with grips to work certain muscle groups.

27. **A)** **Correct.** The sagittal plane uses flexion and extension.

B) Incorrect. The transverse plane uses rotation.

C) Incorrect. This would only be true if the lunges were multiplanar.

D) Incorrect. The frontal plane uses abduction and adduction.

28. A) Incorrect. The maintenance phase is only half of the correct answer.

B) Incorrect. The action phase is only half of the correct answer.

C) **Correct.** Action and maintenance are the phases that will require behavior modification tools.

D) Incorrect. Neither of these phases requires behavior modification tools.

29. A) Incorrect. SMR is self-myofascial release.

B) Incorrect. Foam rolling is self-myofascial release.

C) Incorrect. Dynamic stretching includes active stretches that do not require assistance.

D) **Correct.** Proprioceptive neuromuscular facilitation does utilize a partner to aid in stretching muscles.

30. A) Incorrect. A machine leg extension is not a closed chain movement; a squat would be an example of a closed chain movement—with one or both legs on the floor.

B) Incorrect. A machine leg extension is not a core movement as it only focuses on one muscle group and a single joint motion, as opposed to several muscle groups and joints at a time.

C) **Correct.** In a machine leg extension, the machine allows both legs to lift at the same time, keeping the kinetic chain open.

D) Incorrect. A machine leg extension focuses on leg extension, which is a movement that falls in the sagittal plane of motion.

31. A) Incorrect. Exercise advice is within a personal trainer's scope of practice.

B) Incorrect. A personal trainer's scope of practice includes providing advice on stretching.

C) Incorrect. Providing advice on general health matters is within a personal trainer's scope of practice.

D) **Correct.** Providing nutrition advice does not fall within a personal trainer's scope of practice unless the trainer has additional certification in nutrition.

32. **A)** **Correct.** Muscular power exercises that involve jumping increase the stress placed on the joints from impact and should be avoided.

B) Incorrect. Muscular endurance exercises will benefit obese individuals and cause little joint stress.

C) Incorrect. Muscular strength training benefits obese clients and does not necessarily cause excessive joint stress.

D) Incorrect. Muscular hypertrophy exercises will help to reduce body fat and increase lean mass, overall decreasing body weight and reducing stress.

33. A) **Correct.** A static postural assessment cannot provide information about a client's heart health.

B) Incorrect. A static postural assessment can provide information about joint misalignment.

C) Incorrect. A static postural assessment can provide information about proper muscle length.

D) Incorrect. A static postural assessment can provide information about possible muscular dysfunction.

34. A) Incorrect. The bench press is general and not very specific to the sport of basketball. It may be used during the very early stages of resistance training.

B) Incorrect. The leg press is a stabilized movement that limits core involvement making it a poor choice for a basketball player.

C) **Correct.** The plyometric squat jump is perfect for basketball players' peak performance because it is specific and will help to increase their jumping capabilities. The movement is used over and over in the course of a game of basketball.

D) Incorrect. Rotator cuff exercises may be helpful in rehabilitation from shoulder injuries; however, it is not the most beneficial exercise for peak performance.

35. A) Incorrect. The single-leg windmill is a balance move and not a direct regression for the ball crunch.

B) Incorrect. The full range of motion in a sit-up does not make this a direct regression.

C) **Correct.** Taking away the controlled instability of the ball makes the abdominal crunch the regression.

D) Incorrect. The primary mover for the rotation is the oblique muscles.

36. A) **Correct.** This is not a movement compensation for the single-leg squat.

B) Incorrect. This is a movement compensation for the single-leg squat.

C) Incorrect. This is a movement compensation for the single-leg squat.

D) Incorrect. This is a movement compensation for the single-leg squat.

37. A) Incorrect. The theory indicates six distinct stages of change.

B) Incorrect. The stages are specific, not generalized.

C) **Correct.** There are six distinct stages of change to indicate progressions.

D) Incorrect. There are six stages, not two.

38. A) Incorrect. This is a safe training design that limits the chances of overuse injuries.

B) **Correct.** Rapid progression or training too frequently can cause overuse injuries.

C) Incorrect. Training only one day per week for thirty minutes is unlikely to cause an overuse injury if the intensity is appropriate.

D) Incorrect. Resistance training programs focused on muscular balance help prevent overuse injuries.

39. A) Incorrect. Due to the lack of conditioning the opposite may be true.

B) **Correct.** Because novice clients lack conditioning, they may require more frequent and longer rest periods than advanced clients do.

C) Incorrect. Rest periods should be taken between exercises of the same muscle group and sets of the same exercise.

D) Incorrect. Rest periods should be taken between exercises of the same muscle group and sets of the same exercise.

40. A) Incorrect. PNF increases flexibility and can decrease strength and power performance, so it should be done at the end.

B) Incorrect. PNF should not be done during resistance training as it can have deleterious effects on strength and power.

C) Incorrect. PNF can cause decreased strength and power and can have a negative effect on running or other cardiovascular techniques.

D) **Correct.** PNF stretching should be saved for the end of the workout to improve flexibility.

41. A) Incorrect. Clients should be encouraged to exercise at a comfortable pace based on their assessments.

B) Incorrect. Not all clients will enjoy more difficult workouts; this is highly variable.

C) Incorrect. The best way to ensure the client is getting good value is to make sure the client is exercising in a healthy and effective manner and not always doing a high-intensity workout.

D) **Correct.** Monitoring intensity is a means of reducing risks associated with exercise.

42. A) **Correct.** Active listening uses both verbal and non-verbal communication.

B) Incorrect. Body language is non-verbal communication.

C) Incorrect. Hopefully the trainer is empathetic and building a rapport with the client, but neither of these would be possible without verbal and non-verbal communication, so this is not the best answer. It is certain that verbal and non-verbal communication are occurring during active listening.

D) Incorrect. These are categories of exercises, not communication.

43. A) **Correct.** The trainer should increase the difficulty of the exercise by implementing a progression of the same exercise.

B) Incorrect. A regression would have the opposite effect, decreasing the chances of reaching fitness goals.

C) Incorrect. Stopping exercise after mastering a particular technique will not help the client reach their goals. New goals should be set and achieved.

D) Incorrect. Although a totally new workout may give the client some variety, it will be more difficult to see training progress than simply implementing a progression of the same exercise.

44. A) **Correct.** Fire alarms are typically linked directly to emergency authorities, so the response will be fast.

B) Incorrect. The appropriate personnel may not hear a shout for help.

C) Incorrect. Calling a friend creates an additional step in alerting emergency personnel and will increase the response time.

D) Incorrect. Email is not always readily available and will increase the response time.

45. A) Incorrect. This is too many repetitions and may cause fatigue before beginning.

B) Incorrect. This is not enough repetitions to adequately warm up the client.

C) Incorrect. This is a broad range and still too many repetitions, potentially fatiguing the client.

D) **Correct.** About five repetitions per warm-up exercise is adequate.

46. A) **Correct.** Cueing involves the use of specific movements and words as outlined in this definition.

B) Incorrect. This definition does not apply to exercise.

C) Incorrect. Phrasing does not include using these actions.

D) Incorrect. This is not the definition of sign language.

47. **A)** **Correct.** The pectoral muscles make up the chest.

    B) Incorrect. The rhomboid muscles make up the mid back.

    C) Incorrect. The hamstring muscle is on the back of the leg.

    D) Incorrect. The gluteus muscles form the buttocks.

48. A) Incorrect. The transversus abdominis are stabilizing muscles.

    B) **Correct.** The latissimus dorsi is the prime mover for the lateral pulldown.

    C) Incorrect. The anterior deltoids are synergistic muscles for the lateral pulldown.

    D) Incorrect. The legs are not a focus in a lateral pulldown.

49. A) Incorrect. Resistance training improves strength.

    B) Incorrect. Aerobic training improves cardiovascular fitness.

    C) **Correct.** Clients who enjoy their training programs have better program compliance.

    D) Incorrect. The fitness assessment helps determine client goals.

50. A) Incorrect. Since the person participates in multiple recreational activities, they would benefit from a variety of cardiovascular exercises.

    B) **Correct.** The mode of cardio for a marathoner should be specific to that event: running.

    C) Incorrect. Exercise for general health benefits will be successful with multiple modes of cardiovascular exercise.

    D) Incorrect. Exercise for fitness improvements does not necessitate a specific mode unless the fitness improvement is in a specific cardiovascular activity.

51. A) Incorrect. This is a set.

B) Incorrect. This is not the definition of a repetition.

C) Incorrect. This is not the definition of a repetition.

D) **Correct.** The performance of an exercise one time through its full range of motion is a repetition.

52. **A)** **Correct.** Performing an exercise without compensation means the client is in the autonomous stage of learning.

    B) Incorrect. This is the first stage of learning associated with extreme difficulty during the task.

    C) Incorrect. This is not one of the stages of learning.

    D) Incorrect. This is the second stage of learning associated with minor movement compensations, but the client is beginning to correct technique.

53. **A)** **Correct.** Viewing from three angles will allow the personal trainer to observe gross deviations of alignment and asymmetries.

    B) Incorrect. The personal trainer should observe movement in all planes.

    C) Incorrect. Each client will move differently, but the primary objective is to observe gross deviations during movement.

    D) Incorrect. Holding the body during stance is a static assessment.

54. A) Incorrect. Progression is not the correct term.

    B) **Correct.** There are typically rest periods between sets and exercises in a workout.

    C) Incorrect. Range of motion is not the correct term.

    D) Incorrect. Neither term is correct.

55. A) Incorrect. It is more appropriate to work opposing muscles on a superset. These exercises use the same primary muscles.

    B) Incorrect. It is more appropriate to work opposing muscles on a superset.

C) **Correct.** A push-and-pull or pull-and-push superset is most appropriate.

D) Incorrect. Both of these exercises are push exercises working the same primary muscles.

56. A) Incorrect. The glutes are a synergist in a cable rotation.

B) **Correct.** The obliques are the agonist in a cable rotation.

C) Incorrect. The biceps brachii is not a mover in a cable rotation.

D) Incorrect. The trapezius is a stabilizer in a cable rotation.

57. A) Incorrect. This is a proper body cue.

B) Incorrect. This is a proper body cue.

C) Incorrect. This is a proper body cue.

D) **Correct.** The knees must be soft and agile to move the legs; knees cannot be locked.

58. **A)** **Correct.** The first transition period occurs between the preparatory period and competition period.

B) Incorrect. The second transition period occurs after the competition period, not before it.

C) Incorrect. There is no additional transition period between the competition period and second transition period.

D) Incorrect. The first transition period does not typically occur that early in a periodization.

59. A) Incorrect. This is for development of muscular strength.

B) Incorrect. This is for development of muscular endurance.

C) Incorrect. This will also develop muscular endurance.

D) **Correct.** The repetition range for muscular hypertrophy is eight to twelve repetitions.

60. A. Incorrect. Interval is the incorrect term.

B. Incorrect. Fitness and interval are incorrect terms.

C. Incorrect. Extracurricular is the incorrect term.

D. **Correct.** The acronym is correct.

61. A) Incorrect. The arms falling forward is seen from the lateral view.

B) Incorrect. An excessive forward lean is seen from the lateral view.

C) Incorrect. The lower back arching is seen from the lateral view.

D) **Correct.** The knees moving inward is seen from the anterior view.

62. A) Incorrect. Linear periodization does not implement three different muscular training phases in a microcycle.

B) **Correct.** This is an example of an undulating microcycle.

C) Incorrect. Regression refers to a decrease in exercise difficulty due to physical limitations.

D) Incorrect. The program is not necessarily dangerous if the client has been properly progressed.

63. A) Incorrect. This number is too high.

B) Incorrect. This number is too high.

C) Incorrect. The client could potentially be losing too much or too little, depending on their goals and weight-loss methods.

D) **Correct.** This is a healthy, achievable, and sustainable weight-loss goal for one week.

64. A. Incorrect. Increased lactate threshold is a long-term effect of anaerobic cardiovascular exercise.

B. Incorrect. Type II muscle fiber recruitment is a long-term effect of anaerobic cardiovascular exercise.

C) **Correct.** Both heart rate and respiration rate should increase during aerobic and anaerobic cardiovascular exercise.

D) Incorrect. Type I muscle fiber recruitment is a long-term effect of aerobic cardiovascular exercise.

65.
A) Incorrect. Supporting the wrists is not as safe as supporting the elbows.

B) Correct. Supporting the elbows is most effective for safety.

C) Incorrect. There is no need to support the neck for this exercise.

D) Incorrect. This is not a back-loaded exercise.

66.
A) Incorrect. The sled is an implement for resisted sprint training.

B) Incorrect. The kettlebell is not used in any speed training technique.

C) Correct. The bungee cord is used to propel the runner forward, assisting her in building her speed.

D) Incorrect. The parachute is a tool for resisted sprint training.

67.
A) Incorrect. The bench press test may not be appropriate for prenatal clients. In some situations, prenatal clients should avoid exercises in the supine position after they are twelve weeks into their pregnancy.

B) Incorrect. The single squat may not be appropriate for prenatal clients as their center of gravity has changed due to pregnancy.

C) Correct. The gait assessment would be the most appropriate assessment due to its low intensity.

D) Incorrect. The forty-yard dash would not be appropriate as it measures maximal speed.

68.
A) Correct. A straight-leg deadlift is a more controlled hip hinge exercise than a kettlebell swing.

B) Incorrect. A box jump is an explosive hip flexion exercise.

C) Incorrect. A single-arm swing is a kettlebell swing using one arm, which is considered a progression.

D) Incorrect. A front raise is a shoulder exercise, not a hip and core exercise.

69.
A) Correct. This would be an effective cooldown protocol.

B) Incorrect. Collapsing on the floor in exhaustion risks the blood pooling and delayed onset muscle soreness.

C) Incorrect. Cooldowns should only involve body weight.

D) Incorrect. Static stretching or foam rolling should follow a session of lower intensity cardio.

70.
A) Incorrect. Setting reasonable goals to inhibit the possibility of unreasonable results cannot be considered self-monitoring.

B) Correct. Setting reasonable and attainable goals is an example of cognitive coping.

C) Incorrect. The description provided is not an example of rewarding.

D) Incorrect. Setting reasonable and attainable goals is positive, and is not an example of negative reinforcement.

71.
A) Incorrect. Steady-state cardiovascular training does little to improve lactate threshold.

B) Incorrect. Maximal strength resistance training helps improve muscular strength.

C) Incorrect. Muscular power training helps develop speed but not lactate threshold.

D) Correct. Sprint interval training will help to improve lactate threshold.

72.
A) Incorrect. Cycling is effective at developing cardiovascular fitness.

B) Correct. A fall during road cycling could have catastrophic results for the unborn baby and for the mother. The risks with this activity are too high.

C) Incorrect. The intensity is not necessarily too high and is based on the client's training level.

D) Incorrect. The intensity level can be increased to meet the goals of the client.

73.
A) Incorrect. This repetition range is too low for light loads.

B) Incorrect. This repetition range is too low for light loads.

C) Incorrect. This repetition range is too low for light loads.

D) **Correct.** For short rest periods and light loads, fifteen repetitions are appropriate.

74. **A)** **Correct.** Increases in training load are associated with an obligatory decrease in volume to avoid overuse or overtraining.

B) Incorrect. Decreasing loads are associated with increasing volumes.

C) Incorrect. Maintaining load with a decrease in volume will reduce the chances of the program causing a progressive overload on the muscles. The client won't get the desired results.

D) Incorrect. Both training variables should change when either of them changes.

75. A) Incorrect. A supine position requires the body to be totally flat.

B) Incorrect. A sitting position is not the correct starting position.

C) **Correct.** In a semi-supine position, body is face up on the floor with the knees bent and feet planted on the floor.

D) Incorrect. In a prone position, the body is lying face down.

76. A) Incorrect. Sand is not used during the balance error scoring system.

B) Incorrect. Water is not used during the balance error scoring system.

C) Incorrect. A balance beam is not used during the balance error scoring system.

D) **Correct.** A foam pad is used to increase the difficulty of the task of balancing.

77. A) Incorrect. This is not the correct representation of the CEC acronym.

B) **Correct.** CEC stands for continuing education credit.

C) Incorrect. The CEC acronym does not stand for collective exercise collaboration.

D) Incorrect. Care education collective is an incorrect representation of the acronym.

78. A) Incorrect. Stretch-release is the principle of static stretching.

B) **Correct.** In hold-relax, the stretching partner holds the stretch for 30 seconds and then allows the muscle to relax briefly before stretching again.

C) Incorrect. Relax-breathe is not a stretching sequence.

D) Incorrect. Contract-contract is not a stretching sequence.

79. **A)** **Correct.** The push-up test is used to assess the stability of the muscular endurance of the upper body.

B) Incorrect. The three-minute step test is a cardiorespiratory assessment.

C) Incorrect. The overhead squat test is used to assess dynamic movement and flexibility.

D) Incorrect. The barbell squat test is used to assess lower body strength.

80. A) Incorrect. Although this is positive body language, it might not be an appropriate response.

B) Incorrect. Hugging is one type of empathetic body language, but it might not be an appropriate response to the client's statement.

C) Incorrect. This would be a negative response to a client.

D) **Correct.** Repeating key elements of a client's statement indicates active listening.

81. A) Incorrect. Though some fitness websites may list emergency action plans, an appropriate resource with the governing rules and regulations is more credible.

B) Incorrect. Fitness professionals may have different plans set in place for one facility or place of work, and the information will vary for every individual.

C) **Correct.** The US Department of Labor website lists the minimum requirements for an employer's facility emergency action plan. Various factors will increase the regulations each employer will follow, but the employer's action plan must at least meet the minimum requirements.

D) Incorrect. Local business action plans will vary based on the company size and number of employees. Additionally, these companies may not be following the government rules and regulations and could be subject to litigation themselves. It is best to go straight to the source.

82. A) Incorrect. This will not give the personal trainer an indication of an individual's general cardio health and overall fitness level.

B) Incorrect. This will not give the personal trainer an indication of an individual's general cardio health and overall fitness level.

C) Incorrect. This will not give the personal trainer an indication of an individual's general cardio health and overall fitness level.

D) **Correct.** This is a good indicator of an individual's general cardio health and overall fitness level.

83. A) **Correct.** Exercises that allow foot or hand movement keep the kinetic chain open, usually using a weight machine.

B) Incorrect. Exercises that load the spine are classified as structural.

C) Incorrect. Exercises that keep either feet or hands at a fixed point are closed kinetic chain exercises; they close the kinetic chain.

D) Incorrect. Exercises that rely on a partner to stretch the limbs are PNF stretches (proprioceptive neuromuscular facilitation).

84. A) **Correct.** This is the correct descriptor of the preparation phase.

B) Incorrect. In the contemplation phase, the participant has decided not to be stuck in the same unhealthy rut.

C) Incorrect. In the action phase, the participant has reached the goal and will continue to change as part of his or her lifestyle.

D) Incorrect. Initiation does not occur during termination.

85. A) Incorrect. Outdoor temperatures may be extreme and cause issues with overheating.

B) Incorrect. Exercising in cold temperatures can cause issues with thermoregulation as well.

C) **Correct.** Proper hydration is important because it helps children and adolescents to thermoregulate their body temperatures.

D) Incorrect. Exercise indoors can involve extreme temperatures as well.

86. A) **Correct.** The balance error scoring system requires the use of a spotter since the eyes are closed during portions of the test.

B) Incorrect. The single-leg squat test does not require a spotter.

C) Incorrect. The star excursion balance test does not require a spotter since the eyes remain open during the assessment.

D) Incorrect. The overhead squat test does not require a spotter since both feet remain on the ground.

87. A) Incorrect. This would be an antagonist muscle.

B) Incorrect. This is not a muscle descriptor.

C) **Correct.** This describes a synergist muscle.

D) Incorrect. This would describe the prime mover's motion.

88. A) Incorrect. The A is incorrect.

B) Incorrect. The S is incorrect.

C) **Correct.** SMART goals are specific, measurable, action-oriented, realistic and time-stamped goals created for program compliance.

D) Incorrect. The R is incorrect.

89. **A) Correct.** Exercise specificity is extremely important for improvements in sports. The program should make sure to include sport-specific strength and conditioning.

B) Incorrect. Resistance training every day may lead to overtraining, depending on the sport.

C) Incorrect. This depends directly on the sport in which the athlete competes.

D) Incorrect. Though strength testing is important for many athletes, not all athletic improvement relies on it.

90. A) Incorrect. Maintaining training loads will not elicit the overload effect.

B) Correct. A gradual progression of training loads will elicit the overload effect.

C) Incorrect. Decreasing training loads does not follow the principle of overload.

D) Incorrect. Rapidly increasing training loads can cause overuse injuries and prevent improvements.

91. A) Incorrect. Injury is not an environmental factor.

B) Incorrect. Injury is not in the category of personal attributes.

C) Correct. Injury is categorized as a physical-activity factor.

D) Incorrect. Locus of control is a personal attribute.

92. A) Incorrect. It is necessary to bend the knees to complete a rep.

B) Incorrect. While this is not a part of a rep, raising the toes can be added to a repetition to incorporate the calves.

C) Correct. Locking the knees could cause a serious injury.

D) Incorrect. It is necessary to press into the heels to complete the repetitions properly.

93. A) Incorrect. The term *transitional* does not describe any type of fitness equipment.

B) Incorrect. Cardio equipment is non-portable and focuses on aerobic training only.

C) Correct. Functional equipment is portable and can be used for various types of training.

D) Incorrect. While the stability ball and resistance tubes are used for advanced controlled instability and strength training, a sandbag is used in explosive movements.

94. A) Incorrect. This is the definition of exercise regression.

B) Incorrect. This is called peaking.

C) Incorrect. This is the principle of progression.

D) Correct. A training plateau is when the client is not seeing any benefit from the exercise program.

95. A) Incorrect. It is impossible to peak throughout the entirety of a program.

B) Incorrect. If the client peaks at the start, then there is no goal to reach with the program.

C) Correct. The trainer should develop the periodization to have the client peak just prior to competitions or major events during the season.

D) Incorrect. Peak performance is safe as long as the program does not intend to maintain this high intensity for too long. After peak performance is reached, maintenance training can begin, or an active rest can be taken following the completion of competition.

96. A) Incorrect. The long jump test measures maximal horizontal jump distance.

B) Correct. The reactive strength index test measures the body's reactive jump capacity and the stretch-shortening cycle effort.

C) Incorrect. The forty-yard dash is used to assess maximal speed.

D) Incorrect. The hexagon test is used to assess speed, agility, and quickness.

97. A)   Incorrect. This refers to the training frequency.

B)   Incorrect. This is the type of exercise the client is performing.

C)   Correct. RPE stands for Rating of Perceived Exertion, or how difficult the client feels the activity is on a scale of one through ten.

D)   Incorrect. This is not what the RPE scale represents.

98. A)   Incorrect. A warm-up should be less than moderate intensity.

B)   Incorrect. A power training continuum workout is done at multiple intervals, not a warm-up.

C)   Correct. The warm-up should prepare the body for stretching; it should be done at low to moderate intensity.

D)   Incorrect. High intensity is appropriate for speed training or sprint training.

99. A)   Incorrect. Finger tapping is an indicator of negative body language.

B)   Correct. Tall posture is a positive body language indicator.

C)   Incorrect. Shifting eyes is also a negative body language indicator.

D)   Incorrect. Arms crossed is another negative body language indicator.

100. A)   Incorrect. These are both progressions of the push-up due to fewer points of contact and an unstable surface.

B)   Incorrect. These are both progressions due to the increased body weight lifted and a plyometric jump at the top.

C)   Incorrect. These are both regressions that limit the weight lifted by the arms during a push-up.

D)   Correct. The kneeling push-up is a regression whereas the push-up with feet elevated is a progression.

101. A)   **Correct.** This describes the general adaptation syndrome.

B)   Incorrect. Specificity refers to the program meeting the client's goals through selecting exercises similar to the client's event or competition.

C)   Incorrect. Overtraining is caused by excessive progression or excessive training frequency.

D)   Incorrect. Progression is used to elicit the effects of general adaptation syndrome.

102. A)   **Correct.** It is good practice to be well protected against injury, defamation, and negligence.

B)   Incorrect. This is not necessary for a personal trainer unless the trainer wants to teach group fitness.

C)   Incorrect. A trainer at a gym should not need to buy additional equipment.

D)   Incorrect. A trainer does not need a social media account.

103. A)   **Correct.** This is an observed compensation.

B)   Incorrect. This is an observed compensation during an overhead squat.

C)   Incorrect. This is not considered a compensation during the gait assessment.

D)   Incorrect. This is not considered a compensation during the gait assessment.

104. A)   Incorrect. Plyometrics is high intensity training that can be done in short bursts.

B)   Incorrect. This lengthens muscles and doesn't usually elevate heart rate enough for aerobic endurance training.

C)   Incorrect. Core training is a type of bodyweight resistance training, utilizing slow and controlled movement.

D)   Correct. Circuit training can use various exercises in a continuous sequence with minimal rest causing an elevated heart rate for an extended period.

105. A)   Incorrect. Dynamic stretching helps to improve muscle elasticity and blood flow prior to exercise.

B)   Correct. Static stretching elicits an elongation of the muscle through a static holding of a stretch.

C) Incorrect. Self-myofascial release involves using tools to compress adhesions in the fascia that surrounds muscle bodies.

D) Incorrect. The dynamic warm-up does not involve static stretching to elongate muscle.

106. A) Incorrect. The client needs a physician's clearance since the assessment involves exercising.

B) Correct. The client should obtain a physician's clearance to participate in an exercise program that incorporates that joint.

C) Incorrect. This could lead to potential injury or muscular imbalances.

D) Incorrect. The client could be injured without supervision or advice, and should be instructed to ask a physician how to proceed.

107. A) Incorrect. Vocal tone is non-verbal and words are verbal.

B) Incorrect. Body language is non-verbal and singing skills are neither verbal nor non-verbal.

C) Correct. Vocal tone and body language are both types of non-verbal communication.

D) Incorrect. Words are verbal communication and body language is non-verbal.

108. A) Incorrect. Posterior pelvic tilt is characterized by a posterior tilt of the pelvis.

B) Incorrect. Lower crossed syndrome is characterized by an anterior tilt of the pelvis.

C) Correct. One of the characteristics of pronation distortion syndrome is flattening of the feet.

D) Incorrect. Upper crossed syndrome is characterized by a forward head position and rounded shoulders.

109. A) Incorrect. Fitness professionals will benefit more from a BLS course that also includes AED and first aid.

B) Incorrect. Fitness professionals will benefit more from a BLS course that also includes first aid and CPR.

C) Correct. BLS classes for fitness professionals should include first aid, CPR, and AED training.

D) Incorrect. Evaluating cardiac arrhythmias is beyond the scope of most certified personal training settings.

110. A) Incorrect. While these are exercise adherence barriers, they are not considered the most difficult to overcome.

B) Incorrect. Self-efficacy is correct, but not accessibility.

C) Incorrect. Locus of control is correct, but intrinsic motivators is not.

D) Correct. Self-efficacy and locus of control are considered the most difficult exercise adherence barriers to overcome.

111. A) Incorrect. In the precontemplation phase, the participant hasn't even thought of change.

B) Incorrect. In the maintenance phase, the participant has already acted and is continuing this action successfully, being mindful of relapses.

C) Correct. This is the correct descriptor of the action phase.

D) Incorrect. In the preparation phase, the participant is planning to act within a month.

112. A) Incorrect. A muscle knot causes muscle imbalance.

B) Correct. Muscle imbalances create tightness around joints, leading to poor form and injury if not corrected.

C) Incorrect. Muscle explosion is not a term.

D) Incorrect. The structure of a muscle gives it its function for the body.

113. **A) Correct.** This compensation can be viewed anteriorly.

B) Incorrect. This compensation can be viewed posteriorly.

C) Incorrect. This compensation can be viewed posteriorly.

D) Incorrect. This compensation can be viewed posteriorly.

114. A) Incorrect. This is the assessment that ensures that the content of the tests are relevant and appropriate.

B) Incorrect. This measures whether scores from similar assessments are related to the same outcome.

C) Incorrect. This is based on tests that measure what is intended.

D) Correct. This is the validity that is described in the question.

115. A) Incorrect. This is the last stage of progression the muscles should go through because it is the highest intensity.

B) Correct. A base of muscular endurance should be developed prior to progression to higher intensities.

C) Incorrect. Muscular strength training should be implemented after an endurance and hypertrophy phase.

D) Incorrect. This type of training refers to cardiovascular exercise rather than muscular training.

116. A) Incorrect. Uncontrollable metabolic disease is a relative contraindication.

B) Correct. Symptomatic heart failure is an absolute contraindication.

C) Incorrect. A musculoskeletal disorder is a relative contraindication.

D) Incorrect. A history of heart illness is a relative contraindication.

117. A) Incorrect. This has no bearing on the thoracic spine.

B) Incorrect. This is referred to as lumbar lordosis.

C) Correct. The thoracic spine refers to the mid-back, where the shoulders land.

D) Incorrect. This is referred to as knee valgus.

118. A) Incorrect. This exercise is single joint and not very specific to football.

B) Incorrect. This exercise is seated, the back and core are supported, and the movement is stabilized by the machine, none of which are specific to football.

C) Incorrect. This exercise is seated and the movement is stabilized by the machine, so it lacks specificity.

D) Correct. The push press forces the football player to use the legs and core to produce force to the chest and shoulders, and the athlete must stabilize using their muscles. The exercise is more specific to the sport than the bench press.

119. **A) Correct.** The transversus abdominis is part of the stabilizer muscle system in the core.

B) Incorrect. The hip flexors are part of the movement system of the core.

C) Incorrect. The erector spinae is part of the movement system of the core.

D) Incorrect. The abductor complex is part of the movement system of the core.

120. **A) Correct.** Med ball chops and prisoner squats represent a full range of motion work at a higher intensity, with light or no weight, than a general cardio warm-up.

B) Incorrect. While arm circles could be considered a dynamic stretch, a deadlift is a structural core exercise using a moderate to heavy load.

C) Incorrect. While butt kickers could be considered a dynamic stretch, a hamstring static stretch is clearly a static stretch.

D) Incorrect. Both of these exercises are power moves and are too intense to be dynamic stretches.

121. **A) Correct.** This plyometric exercise is specific to running, and the first transition period should incorporate higher intensity exercises to start building to peak performance during the competitive period.

B) Incorrect. A standard wall sit is not very specific and should be incorporated in the beginning of the preparatory period for beginners.

C) Incorrect. Barbell bench press is a basic strength training exercise that is most beneficial at the beginning of the training program.

D) Incorrect. The triceps kickback is not very specific to triathletes, especially during the first transition period.

122. A) Incorrect. Injuries involving severe bleeding require cleaning the wound, applying a sterile dressing, and possibly seeking medical assistance.

B) **Correct.** RICE stands for Rest, Ice, Compression, and Elevation. This acronym should be followed in caring for sprains, strains, and contusions.

C) Incorrect. Cardiopulmonary issues may be serious and require emergency responders.

D) Incorrect. Chest pain can indicate serious problems such as a heart attack and may require emergency responders.

123. A) Incorrect. This would be a progression of the exercise.

B) Incorrect. This would be a progression of the exercise.

C) Incorrect. This is a different exercise at a similar intensity.

D) **Correct.** A wall sit or wall slide exercise removes the stability required from the core and makes the exercise easier. It is a regression.

124. A) Incorrect. Non-profit organizations often have .org websites, so this will usually indicate a credible website.

B) **Correct.** A .biz website is likely not a credible website for fitness articles and research.

C) Incorrect. Many credible educational websites end with .edu.

D) Incorrect. A .gov address usually indicates a credible government website.

125. A) Incorrect. Body control is synonymous with form.

B) **Correct.** Breath is a key component of exercise technique and lifting heavy loads.

C) Incorrect. Flexibility is important but not necessary when adding heavy weight loads.

D) Incorrect. While a positive outlook is important, it is not an athlete's primary focus when he or she is lifting heavy loads.

Printed in Great Britain
by Amazon

MOUNTAIN
BIKE GUIDE

First published 2006

British Library Cataloguing in Publication Data

Mountain Bike Guide. Nottinghamshire

I. Thompson S.J.

ISBN 1-899043-10-1

Printed in the United Kingdom

Produced by Context Products Ltd
53 Mill Street
Packington
Ashby de la Zouch
Leicestershire
England
LE65 1WN
Tel: 01530 411337
Fax: 01530 411289
Email: enquiries@contextproducts.co.uk

Author Stewart Thompson
Design: John Dunlop
Production: Wesley Ewing

Author Contact Details
56 North Road
West Bridgford
Nottingham
NG2 7NH

MOUNTAIN
BIKE GUIDE

NOTTINGHAMSHIRE

Stewart Thompson

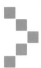

MOUNTAIN
BIKE GUIDE
NOTTINGHAMSHIRE
Stewart Thompson

:> ACKNOWLEDGEMENTS

I have never met Mike Pearce, but this guide would probably have never been produced without him. Until 1999 I only owned one bike, a Dawes Galaxy touring cycle that had a distinct preference for asphalt. It was happy carrying 15kg of assorted clothes, camping gear and food around the Western Isles of Scotland but refused to be ridden over soft or loose ground. In contrast my kids were cycling up kerbs, bunny hopping over logs and attempting all sorts of tricks on a nearby halfpipe. I decided that I needed an off road bike. After 3 months of reading every advert in Mountain Bike Rider, and borrowing all sorts of full sus and hard tail bikes, I got myself a new bike for Christmas. I also got a copy of Mike Pearce's guide to off road routes in the Peak District and Derbyshire. Since then I have ridden the bike through mud which varies from gloopy to sticky, and over rock strewn tracks that mountain goats would be a bit nervous about. However, from working for Nottinghamshire County Council and Nottingham City Council I knew that there were hundreds of miles of potentially good routes on my own doorstep. Since I couldn't find a guide that adequately covered this area I thought I would copy Mike Pearce's idea and produce my own. This guide is the result.

I am especially grateful to all the riders who have vetted the routes and their helpful comments on the production of the maps and the accompanying text. These include Eric Foxley, John Vesey, Grimace Mountain Bikers, Keith Thompson and Slav Kukan.

I would also like to thank my son Thomas Thompson, Ben Shelton, Mathew Cullen, Steven Cullen and Mark Robinson who have accompanied me on some of the routes.

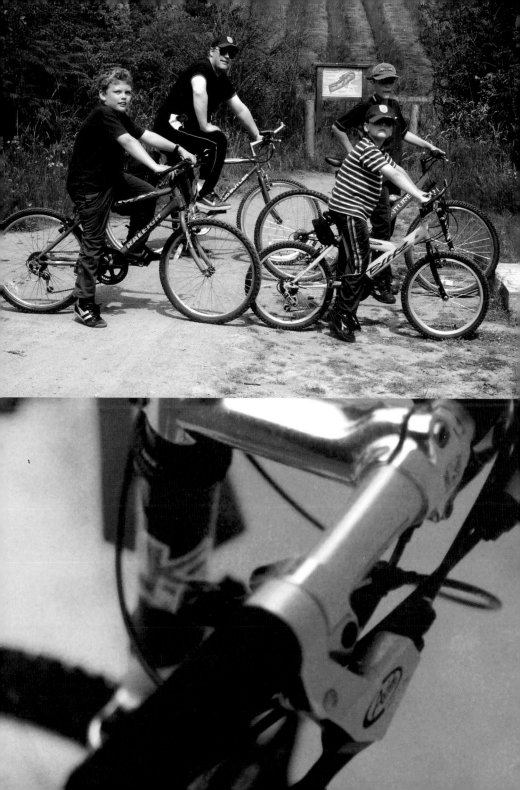

✂ DISCLAIMER

A considerable amount of effort has gone into ensuring that the routes described are both accurate and compatible with the information displayed on Ordnance Survey Explorer maps. However, the author accepts no responsibility for any loss, injury or inconvenience sustained by anyone using this guide.

The inclusion of a route does not guarantee that all sections of it will remain a public right of way. Where there is an absence of signs and well defined tracks the situation on the ground is sometimes confusing and very different from published maps. This guide has endeavored in all cases to stick to the legal right of way. However, where rights of way get ploughed up or unofficially diverted to the edges of fields it is often easy to stray from the legal route. In any conflict with a landowner it is wise to be polite and leave by the shortest route rather than to try and defend your presence. This is best left to the rights of way officer in the relevant Highway Authority.

✂ INTRODUCTION

Some people might climb mountains because they are there, but I produced this mountain bike guide to Nottinghamshire because I couldn't buy one! It contains 22 circular rides, and one linear one, that are predominantly off road. Any on road cycling has been restricted to country lanes that link bridleways or cycle tracks.

All the routes have been selected to provide pleasant cycling in forests, in open countryside, on canal towpaths and on riverbanks. My aim has been to encourage safe, legal cycling that is well away from traffic. The routes range in length and difficulty, but every cyclist should be able to find something within their capabilities. There are opportunities to split some of the long routes and to combine some of the short ones. Decisions of this kind can often be made during the ride so that turning back or extending the journey becomes a matter of personal choice.

✈ USING THE GUIDE

Each of the circular routes has a detailed description and an accompanying map. The maps have been paired down to the essentials to help you navigate easily around a route, and to get a feel of the whole ride at a glance. The scales used vary, but in all cases north is at the top. The key identifies the main features displayed but significant landmarks and buildings are included to help navigation.

The route descriptions provide a brief summary of what you can expect in terms of scenery, wildlife and views. The information on distance, terrain, ride surfaces and suitability for winter use is to help you to chose a route for any occasion. The times are just my best estimates for a reasonably leisurely pace without lengthy pub stops. Your own times are always going to be dependant on how fit you are, how often you stop, how fast you cycle, and how many punctures you get. I would always advise you to cycle these routes in daylight, especially if you are on your own.

The weather can greatly influence cycling conditions on many of the routes. After heavy rain the mud in the Trent valley can clag up your bike in minutes. The softer conditions, increased bike weight, and decreased traction can add hours to a journey and turn a simple ride into a real gut buster. Fixing punctures in these conditions is also a real messy job, and one that numbs your fingers if it is even slightly cold.

It is also necessary to take account of the wind strength. Even a slight breeze can reduce your headway, and I rarely experience the so called wind assisted cycling. All the wind I come across is blowing straight at me whichever way I am pointing.

When choosing a route always consider your own fitness and that of others if you are in a party. There are plenty of easy routes, and most of the longer ones can be broken down into shorter sections if necessary. If you are new to off-road cycling start with a tour of Sherwood Pines, a visit to the Teversal Trails, a trip along the Southwell Trail or a tour around Clumber Park. Build up your stamina and confidence a bit before venturing onto the longer routes. The aim should be to have fun, not to kill yourself.

At some locations you will need to physically lift your bike over a gate, fence or style. There are also some sections that are so steep that you will almost certainly have to push your bike. Although there are very few of these physically demanding situations, you should be fit enough to cope with them.

On some of the routes it has been necessary to include very short sections of footpath to link bridleways and lanes. These are clearly defined on the maps. You are legally entitled to push your bike along a footpath, but not to cycle on it.

⸙ THE RIGHT BIKE

The right bike is very much a case of personal preference. However, for the routes contained in this guide you will definitely need a mountain bike with wide tyres. You can get away with a bog standard frame, but I would recommend a "hardtail". This is a bike with front suspension but no rear suspension. The front suspension gives you much better control on rough surfaces and greatly reduces the jarring on the handlebars. This comfort and stability can greatly increase you enjoyment when riding off road. "Full sussers" take this one stage further by adding bounce to the rear end. They are great fun, and make long distance journeys over rough ground a dream. However, you have to invest a small fortune to get a good one. If you are on a tight budget you can get a lot more for your money with a "hardtail". In all cases avoid the cheap posy bikes that seem to have everything, but weigh a ton even before you put your own weight on them. Remember, that you may have to lift these over a gate or push them up a hill when you are already knackered.

Most bikes come with V-brakes, which are solid compared to the cantilevers on my Dawes Galaxy. Disc brakes can give you more consistent stopping power if you buy good ones, but they push the cost of a bike up considerably. On my own bike I have discs on the front and V's on the back. I suppose I am trying to get the best of both worlds. One great advantage of having disc brakes is that because they are further from the tyres they are less likely to get clagged up with mud. They are also unaffected by buckled wheels or bumps in the rim. If you are buying a new bike make sure it is disc ready so that you can upgrade at a later stage if you need to. I always use mud catchers on both the front and rear of my bike. They are easily detached in dry conditions, but in the wet they are a godsend. I do not like lumps of mud hitting me in the face. Also, I am none too keen on a muddy streak up my back or looking like I have been run over by another mountain biker. I accept that the bike and I will get absolutely plastered on some of the routes if it is raining. However, mud catchers can at least send some of it back to where it came from rather than in your rucksack!

Flat pedals are the best starting point for mountain bikers, and many of us still use them. You can quickly dab your feet down for stability and you can change your foot position slightly if you get uncomfortable. However, for greater efficiency you can switch to clipless pedals or toe clips. This is a matter of preference.

The choice of tyres is a complex subject, but I would recommend a general-purpose go anywhere type. You can get "nobblies" that are more suited to muddy off road conditions, or "slicks" that offer less rolling resistance on tarmac. However, the riding surfaces that most of us travel on are so variable that it seems pointless to get too specific. This is especially true for the routes in this guide.

⊱ EQUIPMENT

A simple day out on your bike can become a nightmare if you get lost, get very cold and wet, have a breakdown, or injure yourself in a fall. For these reasons you need to take a bit of kit, especially on the longer rides. The specified OS map is essential since you may stray from the route and need to orientate yourself. A compass can also help because all the maps in the guide have north at the top.

I don't want to be pessimistic, but you will get punctures. Tyre levers, a pump and a puncture repair kit are therefore essential. A spare tube is often easier to fit than trying to find a leak, especially in cold wet muddy weather. Hawthorn spikes will cause many of the punctures. For your own sanity always run your fingers around the inside of the tyre before fitting a new or repaired tube. You will often find a thorn still embedded in the tyre wall.

I think you should be prepared for a few running repairs, but if you get carried away the combined weight of your tools could equal the weight of your bike. A modern multi-tool like the "Topeak Alien" will fix just about anything that is likely to go wrong. It is expensive, but well made, compact, and light. I regard it as the mountain bikers' equivalent of a Swiss army knife.

A mobile phone is not essential but I often carry one for emergencies, especially when I am on my own. In five years I have never used it in an emergency!

Drinks and food can be bought on some of the routes, but I would always recommend a water bottle and some sarnies. A picnic for me is one of the pleasures of doing these rides.

The clothing you wear and carry is very important. Sunglasses look cool and they are very good for keeping the bugs and mud out of you eyes. A pair of gloves will keep your hands warm and damp down the vibrations in the handlebars. A cycle helmet is a must. It should fit snugly, and the strap should be tight enough to keep it firmly attached to your head, especially if you take a dive over the handlebars. They often make you look a bit stupid, but in a fall they could save your life. Warm waterproof and windproof clothing is often needed when you stop cycling, and in winter it is essential. Modern fabrics are light and breathable so they are excellent for sweaty cyclists.

All the gear can be carried in a small rucksack, or in a pannier that is attached to the rear of the bike. I favor a rucksack because it keeps my gear further from the mud.

⋗ SAFETY

Per kilometer traveled on roads, cycling is 13 times more dangerous than driving in a car. You can reduce the risks by choosing your route carefully, riding defensively, maintaining your cycle, and wearing the right kind of clothing. All of the routes in this guide have been designed to keep a healthy separation between cyclists and vehicles. However, there are locations where you have to cross busy roads, and you should use extreme caution in these situations. When cycling on country lanes it is easy to forget about the other vehicles. Keep to the left, and wear bright reflective clothing so that drivers can see you. At night, you must have lights. Also, reflective material on your clothes and bike is essential. As mentioned earlier, a cycle helmet may save your life.

There is no MOT for bikes, so you have to keep on top of your own cycle maintenance. This involves regular checks of all the moving parts, especially the brakes, wheels, tyres and gears. Brake blocks wear very rapidly in off road conditions, especially where you have long descents on rough ground. Spokes can become slack, nuts can vibrate loose and gears can get knocked out of alignment. Any of these might cause you to fall off.

It is in your own interest to ride defensively and to try and anticipate scenarios that might lead to a crash. For example, you should assume that some pedestrians will not see or hear you and will step out in front of you without looking. When you see a car in a side road, it may pull out in front of you, and at roundabouts this is a frequent cause of injury to circulating cyclists. Drivers often underestimate the speed of a cyclist, and you should cover the brakes if there is the potential for a vehicle to turn across your path.

Off road cycling can be fun, but it can also be dangerous. It is easy to loose control when turning at speed on loose surfaces, and in wet conditions muddy ruts or tree roots can throw you over the handlebars. When cycling near water, especially on narrow canal towpaths, you need to watch out for all sorts of obstacles including fishing tackle, mooring ropes, overhanging branches, collapsed banks, and lock equipment. Swerving to avoid these can lead to a nosedive into the water.

Always give way to pedestrians, and be friendly to them. They share the right of way on all of these routes; so don't hog the bridleways as though you own them. Often you can scare pedestrians to death when they don't see you coming, so slow down and be polite. The continued development of shared pedestrian and cyclist routes is very much dependant on mutual respect, especially from cyclists. However, some cyclists intimidate pedestrians and this gets us all a bad name.

As you would expect, there are horses on the bridleways. To some extent they behave like the pedestrians. They sometimes show no interest in you and at other times get very wary. If they are coming towards you it is best to stop and let them pass. If you come up behind them keep well back until the horse and rider are aware of your approach. Wait until you are sure you can pass without causing the horse to bolt. It is usually possible to exchange a few words with the rider and check out the situation before you go past. Of course all this assumes that you travel fast enough to overtake horses.

Quite a few of the routes go through managed forests. The Forestry Commission actively encourages cyclists, in these areas, but is keen to point out the dangers of forest operations. You must not pass vehicles loading timber until you have been told to do so.

⫸ STAYING LEGAL

A bike is a vehicle and when it is used on the highway the rider must comply with the road traffic laws. It is an offence to ride a bike under the influence of alcohol, to run red lights or to flout the traffic signs. Lights must be used at night, and riders must comply with any cycling prohibitions. This includes cycling on footpaths. Sadly some cyclists blatantly break all the rules in the book. By doing this they jeopardize all the progress that is being made in developing the cycling infrastructure. There is considerable scope for converting footpaths to shared use and opening up more long distance cycle routes, but this will only continue whist the public support the process. If we behave irresponsibly, particularly in the presence of pedestrians, then Highway Authorities will be reluctant to continue investing in cycling. In the papers I do not like to see cyclists stereotyped as lawless loonies who terrorize pedestrians. I would prefer them to be seen for what they are, a complete cross section of society getting exercise by using one of the most environmentally friendly modes of transport you can buy.

⋗ CANALS AND RIVERS

Quite a few of the routes in this guide follow canals or rivers. In many cases you need a British Waterways cycle permit because there is no general public right of way on towpaths. The permit is free of charge and is supplied with a navigation guide, the Waterways Code, and lists of the sections of waterway where cycling is permitted. No permit is required for the Grantham Canal, or the Nottingham Canal, but you will need one for all other canal towpaths. The route descriptions will advise you where a permit is required, and you should remember that one is needed for every bike if you are traveling in a group. The permit can be obtained from the addresses at the back of the book.

⋗ CYCLING WITH CHILDREN

This guide has been written specifically for adults, who are reasonably fit. Some of the routes are suitable for children, but they should be accompanied, equipped with a well maintained bike that is suitable for their size, togged out in safety clothing, wearing a helmet and supervised at all times. Because the age and skill of children will vary, the responsibility for route selection must remain with a parent or guardian. I would strongly advise against taking children younger than 11 on roads. Even if they can handle a bike, they may fail to appreciate the dangers of mixing it with traffic. There are plenty of routes and sections of routes that are traffic free in this guide. This means that you can enjoy cycling with children without having to panic and shout "car" all the time. I would recommend the facilities at Sherwood Pines, Teversal Trails, and The Southwell Trail for any age of cyclist. However, with a bit of pruning down, you can find long sections of suitable off road child friendly cycling within this guide.

Canal towpaths can be dangerous for children, especially by locks, so keep up with your kids at all times, even if you have to bust a gut to do so. This also applies when coming up to a road crossing. Make sure you get their first so that they don't charge across without looking. And one last point, make the journey fun for them, not just fun for you. You could put them off cycling forever if every trip becomes an epic challenge.

TABLE OF ROUTES

Route Number	Route Name	Length in Kilometres	Length in Miles	Off Road %	Estimated Time in Hours
01	Southwell Trail and Farnsfield	31	20	76	3.5
02	Grantham Canal and Cotgrave	27	17	88	3
03	Thieves Wood	23	14.5	93	2.5
04	Trent Valley to Grantham Canal	47	29	84	5
05	Newstead Abbey	25	15.5	73	2.5
06	Nottingham Circular	59	37	73	6.5
07	Trent Valley to Gunthorpe	34	21	62	3
08	Southwell Semi-circle	37	23	71	4
09	Trent Lock	40	25	68	4
10	Towpath Circular	41	25.5	92	4
11	Sherwood Pines	10	6	100	1
12	Sherwood Forest	36	22.5	93	4
13	Clumber Park	27	17	85	3
14	Sherwood Pines Revisited	23	14	98	2.5
15	Nottingham to Langar	65	40.5	77	7
16	Hickling	28	17.5	50	3
17	Belvoir Castle	18	11	67	2
18	Viking Way	21	13	67	2
19	Clumber Park Revisited	15	9	88	1.5
20	Lowdham, Epperstone and Bleasby	29	18	62	3
21	Teversal Trails	23	14	74	2.5
22	Worksop Workout	45	28	78	4.5
23	The Timberland Trail	24	15	75	2.5

Item	Essential	Desirable
Puncture Repair Kit	Yes	—
Tyre Levers	Yes	—
Multi Tool	Yes	—
OS Explorer Map(s)	Yes	—
Drink	Yes	—
Food	—	Yes
Mobile Phone	—	Yes

KEY TO
ALL MAPS

▬▬▬	Route	●●●●●●●●	Railway
▬▬▬	Road	◯	Forest Boundary
▬▬▬	River		
▬▬▬	Track or Cycle Path	●	Lake
▬▬▬	Footpath		
■	Houses	🌳 🌲	Trees
PH	Public House	⋈	Bridge

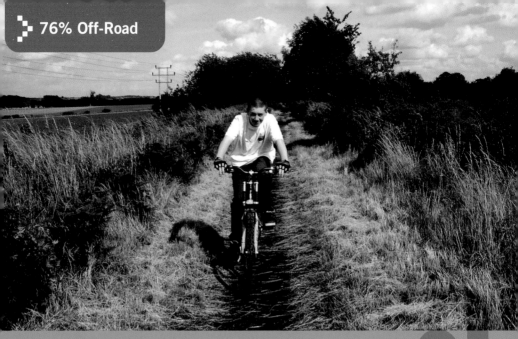

01

SOUTHWELL TRAIL & FARNSFIELD

NOTTINGHAMSHIRE

Route 01

General Information:

Distance	20 miles, 76% off-road
Time	3.5 hours
Maps	OS Explorer 270 Sherwood Forest
	OS Explorer 271 Newark-on-Trent

:> SUMMARY

The start of the route takes in the entire length of the Southwell Trail, which is a disused railway line linking Southwell and Bilsthorpe. The return journey includes a combination of bridleways, and quiet lanes that wind their way through forests and open farmland.

The route is fairly dry all year round, apart from a short section in the woods near Coombs farm and in Eakring Brail Wood. The route along the railway line is flat and the firm surface lends itself to some fairly speedy cycling. By contrast the rest of the route is hilly, very hard going in places, and has a steep technical descent just after Coombs Farm. There are a quite a few places where you have to lift your bike over a style or push it through gloopy mud. Don't let that put you off though since these are the prettiest parts of the route.

:> STARTING POINT

There is free car park at the start of the Southwell Trail. This is situated near the Newcastle Arms public house in Station Road. The OS grid reference is 4706 3544.

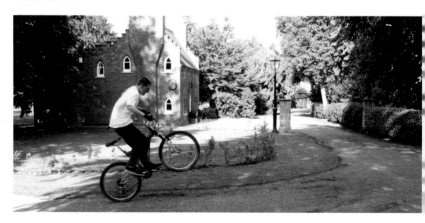

:> THE ROUTE

Cycle along the trail to Farnsfield, which is point 1. on the map. You can always divide the route here, or nip to the chip shop that is just down the lane to your left. As you pass the back gardens of a row of detached houses watch out for a fork in the trail. Bear right to Farnsfield, and keep going until you come to a car park at the end of the trail. Follow the road through the new housing estate and go straight on when you come to the roundabout. The road bears round to the right, and just before you come to the dump you will see a signed footpath on your left. Go over the style, and after 50yds turn right to follow the edge of the dump as far as the wood.

Ignore the footpath going off to your left and dive straight into the woods where you will find a path that eventually becomes a very boggy track. Always follow the ahead route and ignore all the minor deviations or you are sure to get lost. The boggy section is soon replaced by a firm track that ascends steeply to a Y-junction just at the top of the hill. Turn right, and look out for a path that drops away to your left just before you get to the corner of the field ahead of you. This path is regularly used by horses and is often muddy. It descends to the edge of the wood, where you turn right and go to the corner at the bottom. A vast open field should now be visible in front of you. If you look slightly to the right you will see a wood about 100 yards away on a slight hill. There is a bridleway that skirts to the left of this wood but it is often ploughed up and difficult to find. Take this direction, and you will soon see the bridleway sign near the wood. After passing the wood you will pick up a farm track that descends to some kennels. The barking will probably have put the willies up you long before you got here, but it is safe enough to go to the right of the buildings. Follow the lane to the industrial estate and turn right when you meet the minor road. Follow this round the left hand bend until it comes to the A617. Turn left and take the first right into Hexgreave Park. The lane through the park is amazing, but over all to soon. When you come to the T-junction turn right, then first left to take you back to point 1. on the map. Here you can take

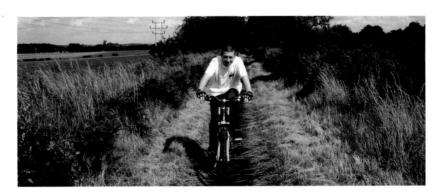

the easy route back, or push on for some real mountain bike adventure. Go over the Southwell Trail and take the road into Farnsfield past the chip shop. Turn right in front of the church, bear round to the left at the next junction, and follow the main road, Longland Lane, out of the village. After half a mile you will come to a bridleway sign on your left. Take the path that follows the left hand side of the field and bear right when a footpath, entering from the left, joins it. Turn right when you reach Coombs Lane. Ignore the first footpath on your left that heads off at right angles to your current direction. Take the second footpath that heads diagonally across the fields just before you reach the farm. Enter the woods after the second field and climb upwards and to your right. Enter the small field at the right of the wood, and climb steeply up the edge of the wood to the gate at the top. Turn left onto the track, which soon becomes a path that descends rapidly down one of the most difficult downhill sections I have come across in Nottinghamshire. The faint hearted should get of and walk, but after lugging you bike up the last hill why not get some pay back. When you reach the lane at the bottom turn left and cycle along until you come to a small group of houses at New Manor Farm. Take the very steep lane on your right which doubles back above the houses you have just passed. When the road starts to level out take the lane on your left that bears to the left of Little Turncroft Farm and becomes a farm track. Follow this across a lane and down into Halam over a small footbridge. Turn left into the village, past the church and straight on at the crossroads to the T-junction with the road to Southwell. Turn right and after 1/2 mile turn left opposite Norwood Park. Follow this lane to rejoin the Southwell Trail and get back to the start.

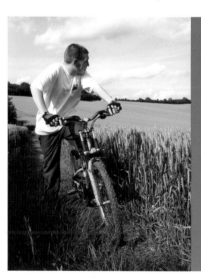

The start of the route takes in the entire length of the Southwell Trail, which is a disused railway line linking Southwell and Bilsthorpe. The return journey includes a combination of bridleways, and quiet lanes that wind their way through forests and open farmland.

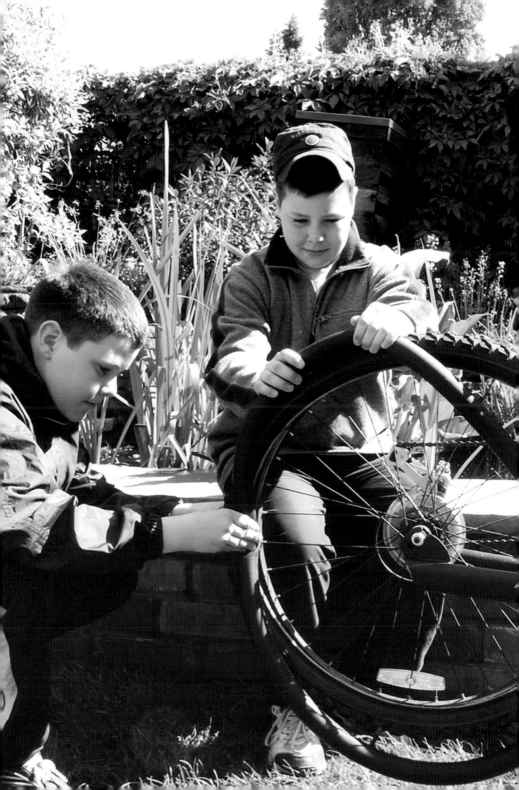

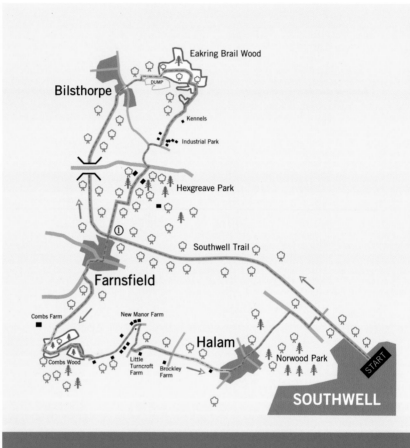

Distance	20 miles, 76% off-road
Time	3.5 hours
Maps	OS Explorer 270 Sherwood Forest
	OS Explorer 271 Newark-on-Trent

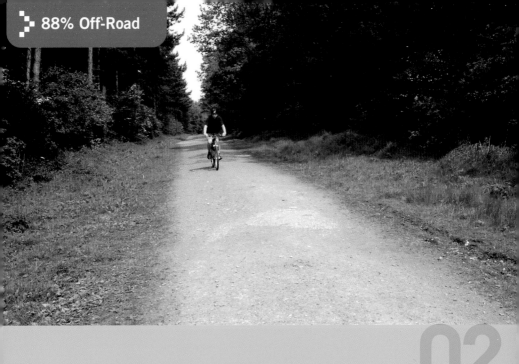

02

GRANTHAM CANAL AND COTGRAVE

NOTTINGHAMSHIRE
Route 02

General Information:

Distance	17 miles, 88% off-road
Time	3 hours
Maps	OS Explorer 260 Nottingham

⊱ SUMMARY

This is a route of outstanding beauty that combines easy cycling along the towpath of a disused canal followed by some demanding off-road hill climbs on quiet forest tracks. The canal still contains water along most of its length that provides a habitat for all sorts of wildlife. You are likely to come across swans and coots sitting brazenly on the towpath yet never see the water rats that disturbingly "plop" into the water just as you cycle past them. The ride through Cotgrave Forest is particularly pleasant on a hot summers day when you get the strong smell of the pine trees and a stillness that gives you that "lazy Sunday afternoon feeling". Most of the route is well drained and the tracks provide a good riding surface, even after heavy rain. However, the first section of Herrywell Lane can sometimes be boggy, especially if you are a 14st rider standing on the pedals and battling to make headway in deep ruts caused by trail bikes and tractors.

⊱ STARTING POINT

There is a free car park on Tollerton Road near the junction with Gamston Lings Bar Road (A52T). The park is clearly marked on the OS map, and is situated on the right just after you have left the main road. The OS grid reference is 4608 3368.

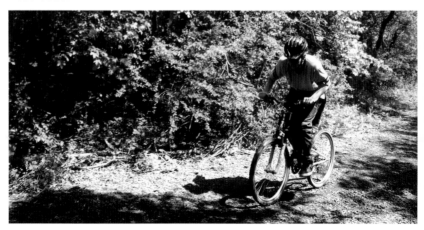

ꞏ THE ROUTE

Cross the road from the car park and join the canal towpath, heading away from Nottingham and the noise of Gamston Lings Bar. Leave the map in you rucksack and enjoy the scenery as you follow the towpath past Cotgrave and under the A46T at Foss Bridge. Keep your head down at this point and try to avoid the drop as you go round the narrow ledge. At Cropwell Bishop the towpath switches to the left hand side of the canal, and soon you will need to be thinking about heading off for some more demanding mountain biking. How the hell do you know where you are though? If you have been observant you will have noticed that mileposts appear at frequent intervals and that the bridges are numbered. After you have passed the 10 1/2 miles to the Trent post look out for Wilds Bridge No. 26. At this bridge turn right onto the very minor road which heads towards the woods you can see on the skyline. Where the road takes a sharp right turn you will notice a wide track which is signed R.U.P.P., although when I passed by this sign had been blasted by a shotgun and was difficult to read! The track is called Herrywell Lane, and the start of it can be very bogy even in summer. Take the track towards the woods and up the gutbusting hill ahead of you. The surface improves here so you should be able to make the crest without dabbing your feet down. Follow the track though the woods and down the hill to the A46T. Wait for a humungous gap in the traffic, the speed of vehicles being very high here, and continue your descend to a small stream. Climb up from here until the track crests, opens out, and meets a crossroads of tracks with open fields on three corners. Take the track on the left that follows the side of the wood, and then descends rapidly into Cotgrave Forest. After the hollow continue on the track until it levels out and then turn right to take the signed bridlepath that forms a wide firebreak through the Forest. Continue for 1/2 mile to the far side of the Forrest and turn right onto the bridlepath signposted to Clipston. This descends to a watersplash, and then goes under some power lines before leaving the Forest to become a farm track thorough open fields.

The track enters Clipston at a right angle bend in a lane near a farm shop. Go straight ahead here and follow the lane down through some sharp bends to the T junction at the bottom of the hill. Turn right, onto Plumtree Road, signposted to Cotgrave. Go through the village entry treatment, past the cemetery and into the village center. At the T junction turn left, signposted to Nottingham, and leave the village on the shared cyclepath. After 1 mile you will meet the Grantham Canal. Turn left onto the towpath and cycle back to the starting point.

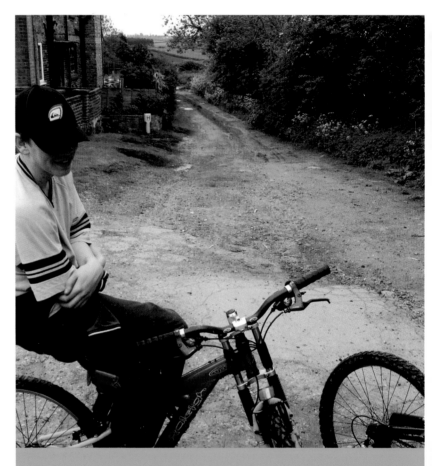

This is a route of outstanding beauty that combines
easy cycling along the towpath of a disused canal
followed by some demanding off-road hill climbs on
quiet forest tracks.

The canal still contains water along most of its
length that provides a habitat for all sorts of wildlife.

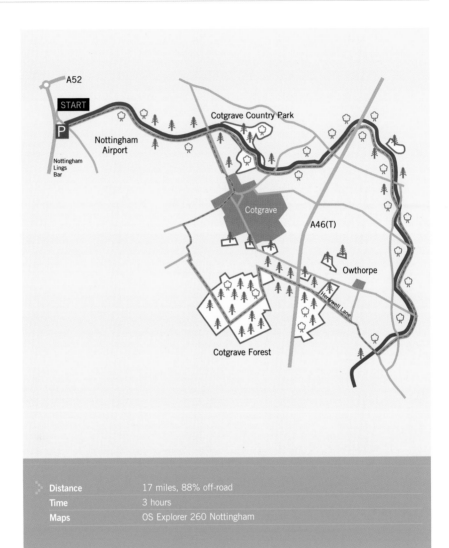

Distance	17 miles, 88% off-road
Time	3 hours
Maps	OS Explorer 260 Nottingham

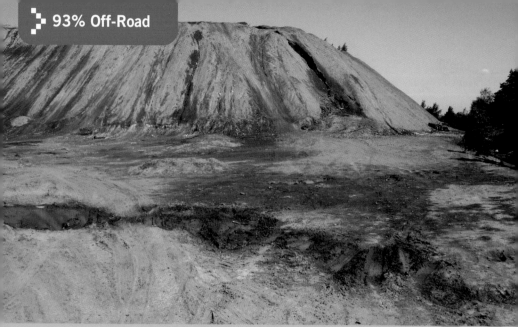

93% Off-Road

03

THIEVES WOOD

NOTTINGHAMSHIRE

Route 03

General Information:

Distance	14.5 miles, 93% off-road
Time	2.5 hours
Maps	OS Explorer 270 Sherwood Forest

❖ SUMMARY

This is a pleasant woodland cycle route that takes in the almost lunar landscape of disued coalmine workings to the east of Mansfield. There is a long section on route 6 of the national cycle network and the adventurous can deviate from the circuit to explore some off road cycling in Sherwood Forrest.

The route is easy going, and is dry at any time of the year. However, there is a short boggy section near Providence Farm where the smell of pigs is beyond belief. The area is abundant with woodland wildlife and birdsong replaces traffic noise for 90% of the journey.

❖ STARTING POINT

There is free car park at Nomanshill Wood on the B6319. The OS grid reference is 4541 3558.

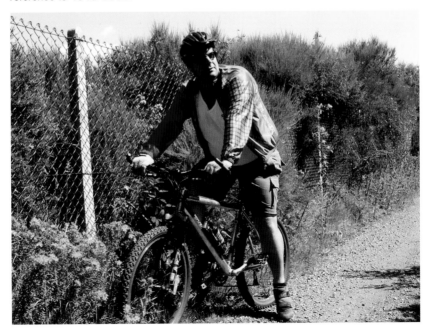

⟫ THE ROUTE

Leave the car park by the signed cycle route which heads away from the road. This follows a broad track through the woods which bears to the left, drops into a hollow and then rises again to meet your return path coming in from the right. Carry on round the left hand bend and then at a point where the marked footpath comes in from your left follow the track to your right. Continue along the track until you come to a distinct footpath heading off to your right. Take this until you come to some large boulders just before you cross the A60. If you get lost in the woods, which is easy to do, panic first and then look for the A60. Use this as a "handrail" to find the road that leads into the new housing estate at Harlow Wood. If you didn't get lost the path would have taken you to this point directly. Don't get too confident though, because there are plenty more woods to get lost in.

Follow the road up the incline until it becomes a broad track through the woods. At the track crossroads, which are at the edge of the wood, turn left, drop down to Old Newark Road, and turn right. It is a mistake to call this a road since for most of its length it is a rough track. Always keep to the right of the houses, and keep a watch out for dumped building materials and garden rubbish. When you reach the main road, turn right and follow the cyclepath to the roundabout. Go around it anticlockwise and take the signed cyclepath on the south side of Rainworth bypass. When you come to a large new footbridge go under it, double back on the footpath and go over the bridge. After descending from the bridge you will come to a wide open crossroads in the woods. Ahead of you there should be a small sandy trail heading up a hill. At this crossroads take the large forestry road to your right. When you come to the T-junction turn left to follow the track up past the huge black slagheap on your left. At the end of this you will find yourself in a coal mining wasteland with black dust everywhere. However, there is a concrete road that runs through it all. You turn right when you reach this road and follow it across two old railway lines before entering Sherwood Forrest through a gap between large boulders at the far side of the clearing. After the boulders turn right through the gate to join route 6 of the national cycle network.

If you want to include a diversion to Sherwood Pines, avoid going through the gate and follow route 6 along the broad fire road that stretches out in front of you. After 1/2 mile follow the red route 6 signs across the railway on your left and enter Sherwood Pines Forest Park. There are several marked routes around this forest, but they will all lead you back to the café and cycle hire shop that is at the opposite side of the forest. If you get lost in this area, which is dead easy to do, find route 6 again and head south.

O.K., so you want to continue with the circuit. It now follows route 6 for about 3½ miles to Providence Farm. Cycle down the edge of the forest with the slagheap on your right. Turn sharp right at the pond, go under the culvert and spiral upwards to join the disused railway line. Follow this under the two road bridges, over a high bridge, and enter Blidworth on Belle Vue Lane, still following the red route 6 stickers that are all over the place. At the main road turn left, and cross over at the shared cycle/pedestrian crossing. Proceed downhill on this side of the road and take the first right which ascends steeply to New Lane. This lane bends to the right and continues rise until it crests near a radio mast. Follow the lane downhill to the T-junction, turn left, and then turn right after ¼ mile at the signed bridleway towards Providence Farm.

Pass the farm and cross the stream before turning left along the riverbank. Pass the small lakes on your left and continue on the path as it enters the woods. The track can be boggy around here and the run off from the pig farm does not help. The smell will give you all the incentive you need to push on quickly to Portland College. Just before you reach the A60, take the path on your right and go to the edge of the buildings. Turn left and follow the path straight over the main road. Keep to the left of the school fence as you enter Thieves Wood and return to the start.

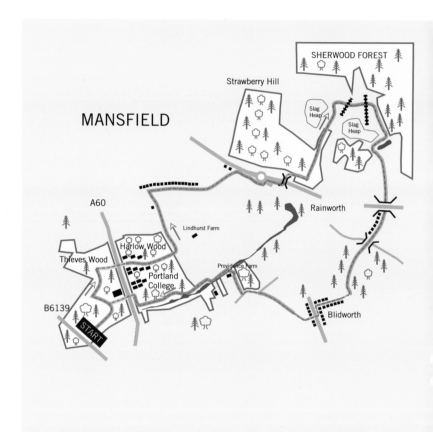

Distance	14.5 miles, 93% off-road
Time	2.5 hours
Maps	OS Explorer 270 Sherwood Forest

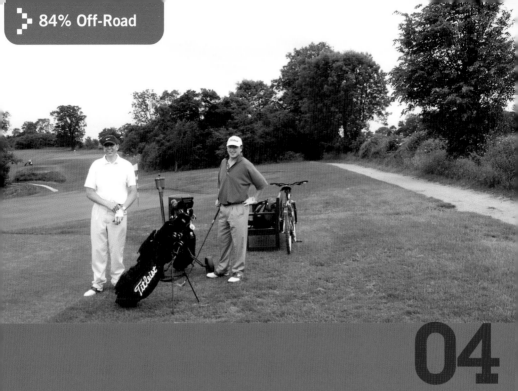

04

TRENT VALLEY TO GRANTHAM CANAL

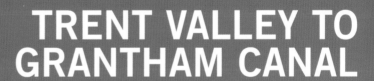

NOTTINGHAMSHIRE

Route 04

Distance	29 miles, 84% off-road
Time	5 hours
Maps	OS Explorer 260 Nottingham
	OS Explorer 246 Loughborough

⊱ SUMMARY

This is a route that follows the bank of the River Trent well beyond the outskirts of Nottingham and across the flood plain to the village of Thrumpton. The route then rises sharply through Gotham Hill Wood and skirts to the south of Nottingham following little used bridleways that link the villages of East Leake, Bradmore, Plumtree and Cotgrave. The Grantham Canal provides the return route to the Trent. The woods in the Trent valley are pretty at any time of the year, but in the summer they provide a shady canopy as you cycle between the river and the very steep bank. Many of the bridleways give wide open views across farmland and the undulating landscape gives a succession of steady climbs followed by rapid descents. The disued Grantham Canal provides an easy ride back into Nottingham and is a good spot for swans at any time of the year.

The bridleway beside the Trent provides good flat riding as far as Barton in Fabis. After this the conditions can get very sticky and mud can clag up every moving part on your bike. There is a really boggy section just after Cuckoo Bush farm, and some unbelievable puddles on the downhill section of Lantern Lane. If you are as happy as a pig in mud then do this route in winter. If you dislike a challenge and like to keep yourself and your bike clean, then only do it in the summer after a prolonged dry spell.

⊱ STARTING POINT

There is free car parking on the Trent embankment near the suspension bridge. The OS grid reference is 4578 3375.

⋗ THE ROUTE

Cross the suspension bridge and follow the shared use cycle path upstream keeping the river Trent on your right. The path rises to the top of a flood bank and drops onto a road. When you come to the Ferry pub turn left and follow the road through Wilford to the traffic lights. Don't cross the main road. Just before the lights there is a cycle path on you right which goes round the building on the corner of the junction. Take this past the restaurant and return to the track that runs along besides the river. When you have passed under the arches of Clifton Bridge take the track to you right. This goes over a small stream and then bears left to follow the riverside all the way to Barton in Fabis. It is frequently signposted as the Trent Valley Way, and you can forget about reading route instructions for a while and gawp at the scenery. At a crossroads of paths go straight ahead and follow the bottom of the bank. Don't be tempted to follow the path on your right that goes to the weir and a dead end.

The Trent Valley Way enters Barton in Fabis by a gate leading onto a minor road. When you reach this road turn right into the village and follow it past the church. Take the second right after the church and look for a style beside a farm on your left. Take the track past the farm buildings, and then follow the path that goes diagonally across a field, dropping to a small footbridge at the far corner. Go over the bridge, turn left and follow the path around the pond and the edge of the field. Resume your direction at a small gate to the right of a hedge, and follow the path across the fields to Thrumpton. Go through the village, past the church and up to the T-junction at Wood Farm. Turn left and after about 150 yards take the track on you right which goes over the A453. This track bears round to the right, then sharp left towards Gotham Hill Wood which should now be directly ahead of you. The track bends to the right behind hillside cottage, and then climbs steeply through a meadow, then woods. As the track crests and leaves the woods go straight ahead into the broad grassy track which descends rapidly and becomes very rough before reaching the road at the bottom. Go over the road and climb up the hill following a very narrow lane to Cuckoo Bush Farm. Just after the farm there is a crossroads of bridleways, and you need to go straight ahead, but do this by switching to the left of the hedge. The route can become very swampy as you approach the woods ahead of you, but it improves rapidly as you descend past the golf course on your left. The track opens up into a road that continues to descend into East Leake.

You join the main road at right angle bend, and follow it round to the right. After 1/2 mile you will come to a roundabout. Turn left and go along Lantern Lane which starts as a road eventually becomes a farm track. After 1/2 mile this turns sharp left, goes past a farm and climbs steeply before descending on a very rutted track to Bunny Lane. When you reach the road turn right past Welldale farm. Follow the road through the left hand bend and even sharper right hand bend. After 150 yards you will come across a rough pull in on you left with two signs pointing across the fields. Take the footpath that goes straight across the field to a footbridge near some trees and a water filled ditch. Cross the footbridge and bear right until you come to a small stream in a deep ditch.

Turn to you left and follow the stream until you come to a bridge where three footpaths converge. Go over the bridge and turn immediately to your left. After 100yards bear right and follow the drainage ditch on your left until you reach a gravel track that crosses the ditch. Follow this to the left for 100yds, turn right for 200 yards, and right again for 100 yards. You will have now gone round three sides of a field, and should take the footpath on your left which heads towards woods on a hill. Keep the hedge on you right, and after 80 yards take the footbridge which goes over the ditch and through a gap in the hedge. Follow the footpath diagonally across the field, over the footbridge, and across a second small field. Turn right when you enter the bridleway and follow it to Syd's bench, which is quite a handy spot to sit and have a snack. Turn left at the bench and follow the track up into Bradmore. You will se the spire of the church on the hill ahead of you.

When you enter the village bear left and go past the church until you come to the end of Far Street. At this point turn left and follow Farmer Street until you come to the A60. Go straight across the road, and follow the footpath for about 60 yards before turning into Mill Lane at the last house in the village. The lane eventually becomes a single track bridleway that goes to the right of, and behind, some modern barns before joining a small lane that descends steadily past Barn Farm. This lane meets the road at a right angled bend near a car park. At this point take the lane on your right which immediately bears left over a filled in cattle grid. Follow the track down the hill towards a house, and at a point 150 yards away switch to the left side of the hedge. You pass the house on a bridleway that descends gently before bearing right up a slight hill and then sharp left under a railway bridge.

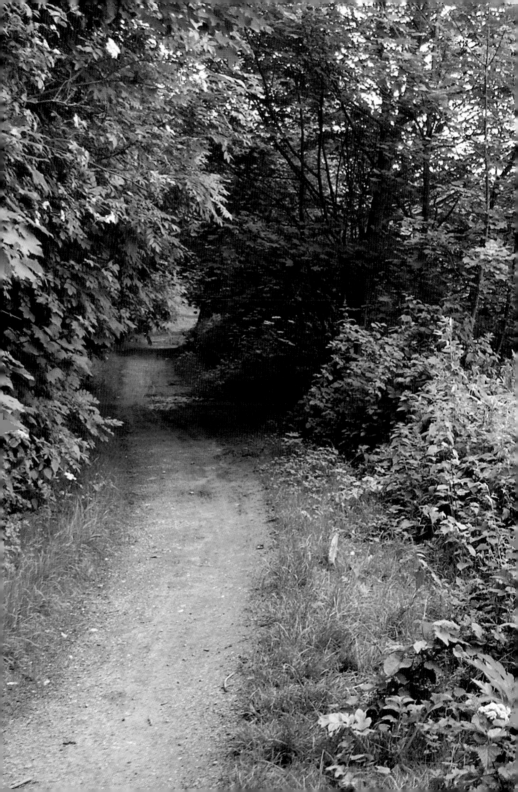

Turn right into Plumtree when you meet the road and turn left at the crossroads into Church Hill. Bear left after you pass the church with the clock tower, and follow the sign for Nottingham. At the traffic signals go straight across and take the first right, which is small a lane signed to Clipston on the Wolds. Proceed to Clipston, where you can link to route 2 in reverse if you are a real sucker for punishment. Those with any sense will continue on the route by cycling straight through Clipston and down the hill on the far side. At the bottom of the hill turn right at the T-junction and follow the sign to Cotgrave. In the center of the village turn left at the Post Office following the sign to Nottingham. Go past the Rose and Crown pub and join the shared use cyclepath as you leave the village.

Follow this to the disused Grantham Canal and turn left towards Nottingham following the towpath on the left hand bank. This path provides good cycling conditions all the way to Gamston Lings Bar a busy, high speed road, on the outskirts of Nottingham. Cross this with caution using the opening in the safety fence just to the right of the end of the canal. On the other side of the road stay on the verge and turn left for 50 yards until you see the sign for the continuation of the canal. Follow this to the right and resume your journey on the left bank. Your next obstacle is a bridge under the A6011 and a gap in the safety fence to get back to the towpath. Here you need to be careful down the steps under the bridge or you will end up in the canal. The road crossing is equally dangerous so leave a big gap in the traffic. The canal towpath gets very narrow for the last half mile and eventually you pop out of a gate near a pelican crossing. Turn right into Rutland Road, go over the canal and turn left at the T-junction. This is also Rutland Road. Follow it to the end and turn left at Trent Boulevard. Just before the signals turn right into Holme Road and pass the playing fields. After passing the adventure play area with a half pipe, turn left to follow the path down to the river. Turn left to proceed upstream under the old railway bridge, past the end of the canal, and under Nottingham Forrest's Trent End. Follow the path that goes down to your right and under Trent Bridge. Continue along the riverside until you reach the suspension bridge and collapse when you cross it to get to the start of the route.

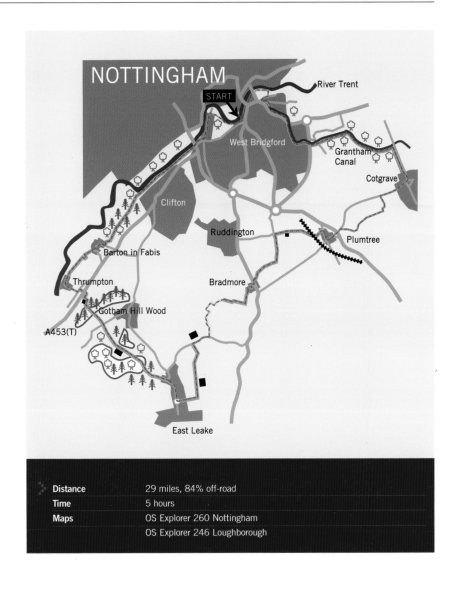

Distance	29 miles, 84% off-road
Time	5 hours
Maps	OS Explorer 260 Nottingham
	OS Explorer 246 Loughborough

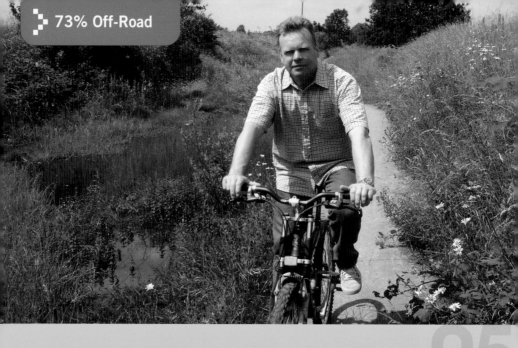

73% Off-Road

05

NEWSTEAD ABBEY

NOTTINGHAMSHIRE

Route 05

Distance	15.5 miles, 73% off-road
Time	2.5 hours
Maps	OS Explorer 270 Sherwood Forest

❯ SUMMARY

This is an interesting route that provides variety in some very undulating countryside. In other words it's hilly and you'll like it. It begins with a fire road through a pine forest that breaks into the open country lanes around Blidworth. It then follows route 6 of the national cycle network to Ravenshead and through the grounds of Newstead Abbey. The return route includes the attractive village of Linby and Burntstump Country Park.

The route is mostly on sandy soil. This means you can even do it in the rain if you're daft enough. The woods are mostly managed for timber production, but nevertheless they still support a considerable amount of wildlife. Birds are abundant along the entire route

❯ STARTING POINT

There is free car park at Blidworth Woods on Longdale Lane. The OS grid reference is 4592 3524.

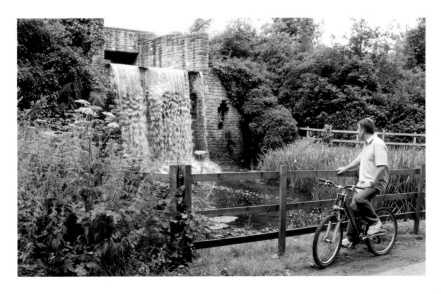

❯ THE ROUTE

Leave the car park on the broad fire road that leads up a steep hill and away from Longdale lane. The blue forestry trail starts in this direction, but within 100yds heads away to the left. It is tempting to take this trail when you see the size of the hill, but your route goes to the top. Follow the roller coaster ride on the fire road all the way to the car park at Blidworth Bottoms. Turn left when you reach the road, pass the stables and turn right onto Beck Lane, the muddy track beside the house. This ascends to Blidworth, and becomes a road as it drops to the B6020. Turn right at the main road and follow it down into the center of the village. As the road starts to rise again turn left beside the chip shop which is just before you get to the traffic signals. Take the lane up the hill, past the library, and bear right onto a track called New Lane. Go past the radio mast and descend to join a road at a sharp bend. Turn left and go down the hill only to find an even bigger one on the other side which goes to a T-junction. Turn right and after 1/2 mile look out for Robin Hood Scout Camp on your left. After the Camp turn left onto the bridleway that descends to Ravenshead where you can follow the route 6 signs through the housing estate.

When the bridleway reaches the main road, go over it to the shared footpath on the far side. Follow this to the right, turn left into Bretton Road and continue to go uphill on Hereford Road. After the crest turn right into Swinton Rise and Right again at the T-junction with Church Drive. Go straight over at Sheepwalk lane and follow the footpath that descends beside Pilgrim close. At the bottom take the Pelican Crossing over the A60 and enter the grounds of Newstead Abbey. Follow the lane around the lake and past the waterfall. Continue on the lane past Abbey Fields Farm and immediately after the gatehouse take the sandy lane on your left that is signed route 6 to Hucknall. This follows the lane for 20yds then turns sharp left onto a disused railway line. Follow this to a roundabout and turn left into the village of Linby. Go past the pub and through the village. After the last house on your left take the footpath that veers to the left along the edge of open fields. This descends to a crossing of the river Leen before rising again to join a narrow lane. Turn right here, and right again at the main road when you enter Papplewick. Go straight ahead at the slightly staggered crossroads near the pub. After 1/2 mile take the footpath on your left, signposted to Seven Mile House. This is directly opposite the T-junction at Papplewick Moor where a road to the right is signposted to Hucknall.

Follow the footpath across open fields, to the right of a farm, and then parallel to a railway line. The path eventually descends into woods before meeting the A60 at some steps beside a railway bridge. Go right over the bridge and stay on the path all the way to the signals ahead of you. Push your bike over the signals to the minor road on your left, and follow this for 300yds before turning right into Sherwood Lodge Drive. Follow the road past the hospital, and take the path on your left just before you get to the Police HQ. This ascends beside the car park, enters the woods and levels out on lane that bears to the left past some rugby fields. Follow this lane to the T-junction and turn left onto the main road. After 50yds turn right down a track past a cul-de-sac sign and follow it past some houses and down the side of a wood. Join the road at a sharp bend and immediately leave it again by turning right into Sansom Wood. Follow the sandy fire road through the wood, bearing to your left as you approach and cross the railway line. Descend to Longdale Lane and turn right. The car park, and start of the route, is just along the lane on your left.

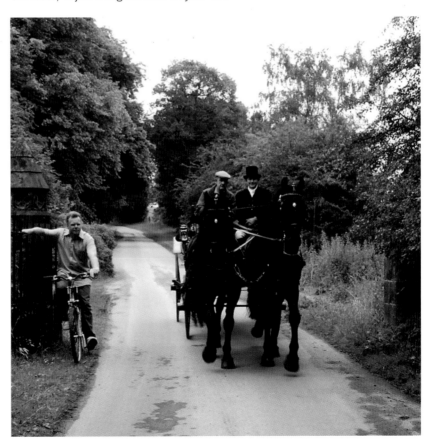

41

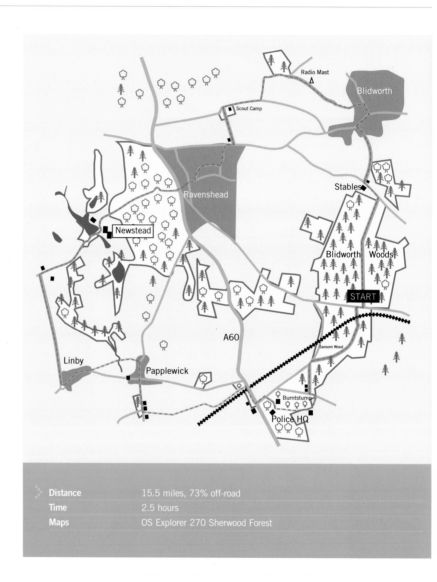

Distance	15.5 miles, 73% off-road
Time	2.5 hours
Maps	OS Explorer 270 Sherwood Forest

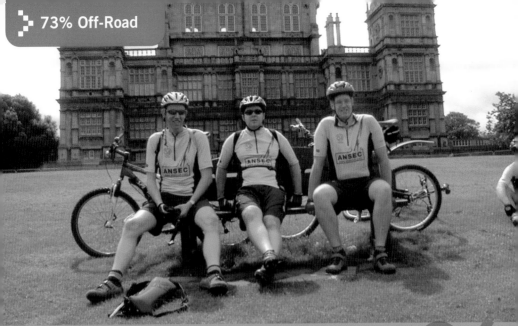

06

NOTTINGHAM CIRCULAR

NOTTINGHAMSHIRE

Route 06

Distance	37 miles, 73% off-road
Time	6.5 hours
Maps	OS Explorer 260 Nottingham

⟫ SUMMARY

This is a ride that takes you on a complete circuit of Nottingham using mostly bridleways, cycle tracks and quiet roads. It is surprisingly rural, given the fact that you are rarely more than 5 miles from the city center. It is also interesting since it takes in Wollaton Park, Nottingham Canal, Bulwell Park, Bestwood Country Park, the Trent valley and Colwick Park. Each of these areas can offer some extended riding for mountain bikers.

The route is fairly flat, especially on the flood plain of the river Trent. However, there are a few steep climbs to the north of Nottingham that come as a surprise after so much easy going cycling. This is a route that can be used in all weather conditions, but riders should be prepared for a couple of muddy sections near Strelley and Burton Joyce. The route cannot be used in the dark since park gates are shut at dusk. It is a long route rather than a technically difficult one. However, halfway round you can cop out to follow route six of the national cycle network all the way back to the start. You can do the rest another day, assuming you recover of course!

⟫ STARTING POINT

There is free car parking on the Trent embankment near the suspension bridge. The OS grid reference is 4578 3375.

❯ THE ROUTE

Cycle along the river Trent embankment heading upstream and away from the suspension bridge. Go past the next bridge on your left and stay on the marked cycle path. Follow this cycle path to the right and go across the road. The route is signed to Lenton. Turn left into the minor road, and after 200yds turn left again to follow the marked cycle lane straight over the main road at the signaled junction. On the far side of the junction turn right immediately into Birdcage Walk. Follow the cycle route round to the left, where it runs parallel to the stream. At the road turn right, go over the railway bridge, continue over the canal, and after the toucan crossing turn left into Old Church Street. Go through the gap at the end, turn right, and use the toucan ahead of you to get across the main road. On the far side turn left, and proceed for 50yds before turning right to follow the side of the stream again. Do not be tempted to go over the cycle bridge, but follow the cycle signs for Wollaton Park. After 200yds cross to the other side of the stream, and continue to follow the track on the left bank beside the hospital. Go straight over the main road using yet another toucan, and pass the old gatehouse which was once part of Wollaton Park. At this point you are on route six of the national cycle network. (N.B. Remember this location if you break the route into two halves and return on route 6) Turn left onto the road after the gap, and follow it to the end, leaving route 6 and following the signs for Wollaton Park. Don't take either of the roads on your right, despite all the attractive cycle signs. Go straight over the ring road using the Pelican crossing, turn left, and then right into Wollaton Park. Follow the lane past the golf club entrance, and through the gate that is locked shut after dusk. Go up the track and arc round to the right in front of the hall, past the red telephone box, through the industrial museum yard, and then sharp right as you leave the buildings to descend to lake. Walk through the buildings please because this is a very popular pedestrian area. You should aim for the right hand corner of the lake, and after crossing the bridge take the sandy track on your right that goes up the hill.

Go through the gates and turn right into Parkside, following this road to the T-junction at the end. Turn left into Bramcote Lane, and immediately right into Glenwood Avenue. Turn left at the end of this road, past the school entrance and right into Fernwood crescent. When you come to the main road go straight on into Grangewood Road which is just offset slightly to your right.
After 300yds, and just before this road turns sharp left, turn right and immediately left into Latimer Drive. After 100yds leave the road to join the Nottingham Canal Trail on your right. Go under the railway bridge, minding your head, over the main road, and then follow the canal towpath to the garden center. Go to the far side of the center to rejoin the canal, but cross the bridge to the opposite bank. At the style turn left and follow the footpath beside the canal on the right hand bank until you come to a large basin. Turn right over the style and take the footpath that follows the hedge to the top left corner of the

field. Go over the double style and turn right at the road. After 200yds turn left into Waterloo Lane following the signed bridleway to Srelley. After 300yds leave the road to enter the signed bridleway on you right. Go through the gate and turn left, following the hoof prints along the left hand side of the fields next to the hedges. At a crossroads of bridleways go straight on and you will eventually go over a horse step before an intersection of five paths and tracks. Take the third on the left that is a farm track that firms up, becomes a lane and bears to the right before entering Strelly.

Turn left and follow the road past the church. At the end of the road continue on the track signed to Swingate that goes over the motorway. At the far side of the bridge turn left and right around the edge of the field before heading away from the motorway. Go over the fields to Swingate, and follow the road that you join as far as the White Lion Pub. Turn right, and at a T-Junction on a bend in the road turn right again into Knowle Lane. Follow this road to the end, past the culls de sac sign, past the park and over the spectacular bridge that goes over the A610. Go down the steep hill on the other side until you reach the main road and turn left. Go straight on at the mini-roundabout, and turn right into Newdigate Street after the zebra crossing. Follow this traffic-calmed road up the hill, past the disused railway line and then turn left when you meet the main road. Go past the Royal Oak public house, and turn right onto the footpath opposite Trough Road. This runs along the side of house No. 54 before entering open fields. As you approach the motorway bear left, go over the style and turn right to cross over the motorway bridge. Just after the bus shelter turn right onto the bridleway signed to Hucknall. After 200yds turn left across the field to the woods. Then go straight ahead with the airfield on your left and the lakes on your right. Go past the isolated houses, and after passing the control tower and the wind soc turn left onto the footpath that runs between the allotments. Go past the end of the runway, the pillbox, and the edge of the golf course. At the corner of the golf course follow the path to the right, passing the 13th T on your right and the large old stable building on your left. Keep bearing round to the right, and go through the car park to the left of the children's playground. Continue down the path in the center of the rows of trees, across the playing fields, and between the two lakes ahead of you. Turn left after passing between the lakes and follow the lake round to the pipe bridge at the far end. Turn right into the woods at this point and head away from the playing fields. As you leave the woods bear left and go through the low point in the old railway embankment. Then drop down to the main road and turn left to the roundabout. Cross over the road just before the roundabout and go straight ahead on a footpath signposted to Bestwood. This path immediately crosses a railway line, and enters a lane that leads you to a main road. Turn left at the road and go under the disused railway bridge. Turn left at this point and take the steps up the side of the bridge. At the top turn left and go over the bridge. You are now on route 6 of the national cycle network. Follow this for 1/4 mile to a point where it joins another cycle route coming in from the left. There is a linked chain sign at this location.

You are now at the halfway point. If you want a fast return to the start follow the route 6 signs through Nottingham and all the way back to the Hospital you passed earlier. For those who are determined to complete this epic in one go, turn left past the sign and after 200yds turn left again where the paths meet. Don't be tempted to go up the reclaimed slagheap, but skirt round it to the left and past the old pithead winding gear. Go over a small stream, and turn right towards the wooded hills. Keep to the broad track, and avoid all the smaller paths. When the track divides, take the steep one on the left and avoid the signed route to Bigwood. The track winds its way upwards through the woods. Where it crests bear right to the T-junction, then turn left onto Woodmans trail that descends beside the fields at the edge of the wood. Go past the toilets, and turn right at the leafy lane to pass under Alexandra Lodge. Follow this lane up through the woods until it crests at a T-junction. Turn left, and then right after the stables. Go up the hill with the horses on your right, and then follow the footpath that descends rapidly between the hedges. Continue on this path until it meets the houses. When you meet the road, follow it round to the left and then down to the Mansfield Road.

Turn right to the signals, cross the main road and straight on into Redhill Road. Follow this over the hill and right at the bottom. When you reach the next junction turn left into Coppice Road and follow it up the hill that goes on for a grueling mile before you come to a mini-roundabout. Turn right to the next mini-roundabout, then left into Spring Lane following the signs to Lambley. After a mile the footpath on the left stops and crosses to the other side of the road just before a sharp left hand bend. At this point you cross the road to follow a bridleway that is signed to Lambley and Burton Joyce. At the radio mast turn sharp right though the gate, and then left at the isolated house. Keep going straight ahead at this point, continuing to follow the bridleway through the gates. Avoid the tempting track that descends to your right. When you meet the potholed lane turn right, and left again just before the lane starts to descend. Follow the track to the isolated house, and turn right just before you get there. The bridleway goes around a field and to the right of the house before descending to track that enters Bulcote beside a church. Turn left at the main road, and immediately right into Old Main Road. Follow this road through the village, over the railway line and past Bulcote farm. Bear to the right, under the power lines and turn sharp right when you meet the wide bridleway that is called Trent Lane. Pass under the power lines again and continue on the track as it firms up and becomes a lane between the river and the railway lines. Go through the gate into Stoke Lane and follow the riverbank to the Ferry Boat Inn. Just after the pub veer to your left, away from the lane, to follow the track along the side of the river. Continue to follow the footpath past Stoke Lock, and immediately after going under the railway bridge, climb up the flood bank and turn right on a path that takes you into the industrial estate and away from the river. You can't miss the path, it is a rubbish-strewn mess beside a concrete molding area. The road you enter is depressing to say the least, and it is aptly named "Road No.4".

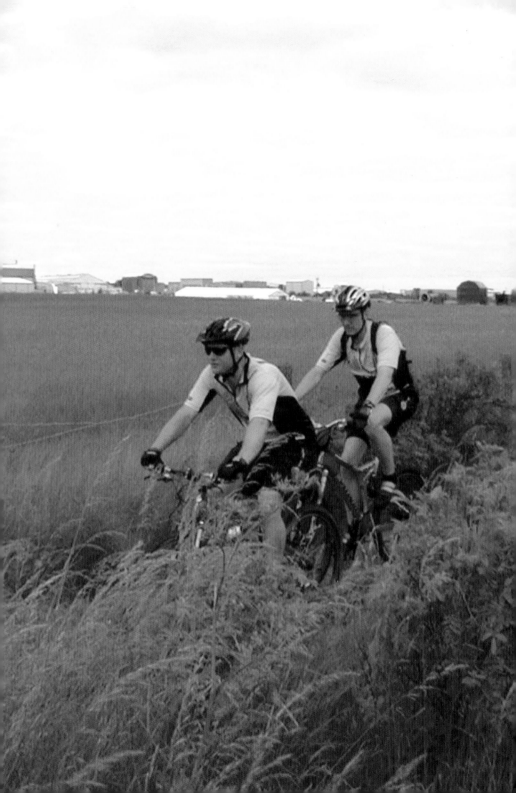

Follow this road straight on for 1 mile through an intensive industrial area avoiding any temptation to turn towards the river because you can't follow the riverbank. I know, because I have tried this myself. The road eventually passes some new housing on the left called Crosslands Meadow. It then turns sharp right. At this point go straight ahead into Colwick Park and take the track on your right when you meet the first lake. Follow this track round to the left, and stick to it all the way through the park. You will pass a bewildering arrangement of lakes and woods, but you cant get completely lost because you are always between the river and the race course. At the end of the park join the road at the edge of the racecourse and turn left. After 100 yards the road turns to the right, and on your left you will find a signed cycle route to Nottingham.
This goes through a small gap, turns to the left and then right onto yet another industrial estate road called Little Tennis Street. At the end turn right, go to the main road and turn left. Go past the roundabout and turn left into Poulton Drive. This is another industrial area. Go to the end of the road and turn right into Freeth Street. Towards the end you will find Lady Bay Bridge ahead of you. Cut through to the main road, and cross it to get to the far side. Now turn left and follow the footpath that takes you over the bridge. On the far side take the steps down to the river. There are cycle ramps on the steps to make it easier to get your bike down. At the bottom proceed upstream along the embankment and past Forest football ground. Keep to the riverside and go under Trent Bridge. Continue on past County Hall until you come to the suspension bridge. Cross this to get back to the start of the route and congratulate yourself on completing a tough circular route around the whole city.

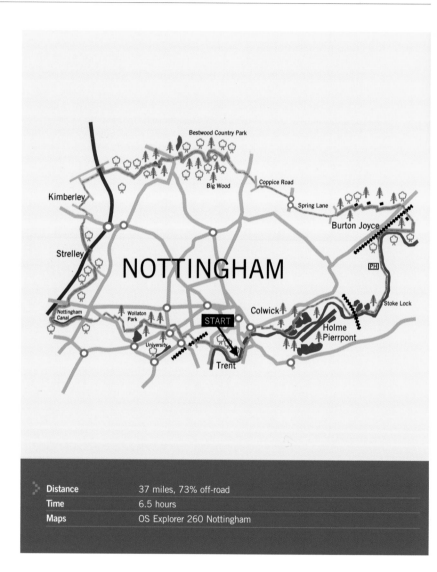

Distance	37 miles, 73% off-road
Time	6.5 hours
Maps	OS Explorer 260 Nottingham

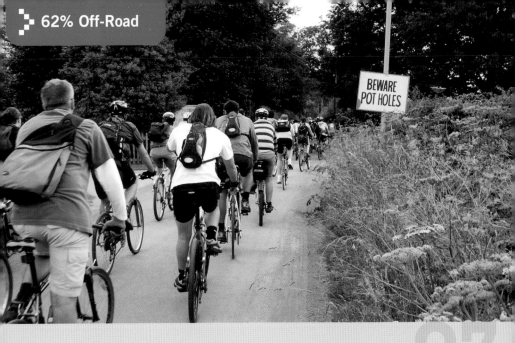

62% Off-Road

07

TRENT VALLEY TO GUNTHORPE

NOTTINGHAMSHIRE

Route 07

Distance	21 miles, 62% off-road
Time	3.0 hours
Maps	OS Explorer 260 Nottingham

> SUMMARY

This is an easy ride that takes you along the Trent embankment from Nottingham to Gunthorpe. On the way out you follow the south side of the river, and on the return you take the north side. There is no public access to some sections of the riverbank, so you have to deviate a bit here and there. However, two of these diversions take in Colwick Park and Holme Pierrpont that are well worth a visit in their own right.

There are plenty of water loving birds along the entire route and you are sure to see a few herons looking for fish in shallow water. At the halfway point you can find a good pub in Gunthorpe, and another one later on at Stoke Bardolph called the Ferry Boat. The route is very flat with good firm surfaces that are pleasant to cycle along at any time of the year.

> STARTING POINT

There is free car parking on the Trent embankment near the suspension bridge. The OS grid reference is 4578 3375.

⟫ THE ROUTE

Start the route by crossing the suspension bridge and turning left to follow the river downstream on the southern bank. Go past County Hall, under Trent Bridge, past Nottingham Forrest Football Club and under Lady Bay Bridge to enter the open fields beyond. Keep to the riverbank until you pass the grassy area in front of the sailing club and enter Holme Pierrpont. Keep following the river past the car park and then join the road that takes you to the start of the white water canoe course. It is well worth the walk along the footpath beside this course since some of the canoeists can handle the rapids with amazing skill. At the end of the rapids go over the bank on your right where you will find the National Water Sports Center lake. Turn left, cycle around the end of the lake, and back on the far side towards the main buildings. Go past the water skiing lake on your left, and when you are one third of the way along the main lake take the track that doubles back up the hill on your left. At the lane beside the gate turn right past the ponds, and follow this over the road humps until you come to a T-junction. Turn Left into Holme Lane and follow this as it degenerates into a muddy track for 300yards. Continue on the lane past Holme farm, under the railway bridge and into Ratcliffe on Trent.

At the main road turn left and go past the church before turning left again into Shelford Road. Go over the railway bridge, continue uphill until you leave the village and then pass a wood on your left. The road descends to a T-junction where you turn left onto a lane signed to Shelford. Follow this lane down the hill, bear right through Shelford and continue until you meet the river again near Gunthorpe Bridge. Go over the bridge and immediately cross over the main road to take the lane that leads down to the pub. At the bottom of the incline bear sharp right along the side of the river to double back under the bridge.

Follow the north bank upstream for 1 mile and take the signed bridleway on your right. This bridleway is called Trent Lane and it cuts out a sweeping bed in the river. Pass under the power lines and continue on the track as it firms up and becomes a lane between the river and the railway lines. Go through the gate into Stoke Lane and follow the riverbank to the Ferry Boat Inn. Just after the pub veer to your left, away from the lane, to follow the track along the side of the river. Continue to follow the footpath past Stoke Lock, and immediately after going under the railway bridge, climb up the flood bank and turn right on a path that takes you into the industrial estate and away from the river. You can't miss the path, it is a rubbish-strewn mess beside a concrete molding area. The road you enter is depressing to say the least, and it is aptly named "Road No.4". Follow this road straight on for 1 mile through an intensive industrial area avoiding any temptation to turn towards the river because you can't follow the riverbank. I know, because I have tried this myself. The road eventually passes some new housing on the left called Crosslands Meadow. It then turns sharp right. At this point go straight ahead into Colwick Park and take the track on your right when you meet the first lake. Follow this track round to the left, and stick to it all the way through the park. You will pass a bewildering arrangement of lakes and woods, but you cant get completely lost because you are always between the river and the race course. At the end of the park join the road at the edge of the racecourse and turn left. After 100 yards the road turns to the right, and on your left you will find a signed cycle route to Nottingham. This goes through a small gap, turns to the left and then right onto yet another industrial estate road called Little Tennis Street. At the end turn right, go to the main road and turn left. Go past the roundabout and turn left into Poulton Drive. This is another industrial area. Go to the end of the road and turn right into Freeth Street. Towards the end you will find Lady Bay Bridge ahead of you. Cut through to the main road, and cross it to get to the far side. Now turn left and follow the footpath that takes you over the bridge. On the far side take the steps down to the river. There are cycle ramps on the steps to make it easier to get your bike down. At the bottom proceed upstream along the embankment and past Forest football ground. Keep to the riverside and go under Trent Bridge. Continue on past County Hall until you come to the suspension bridge. Cross this to get back to the start of the route.

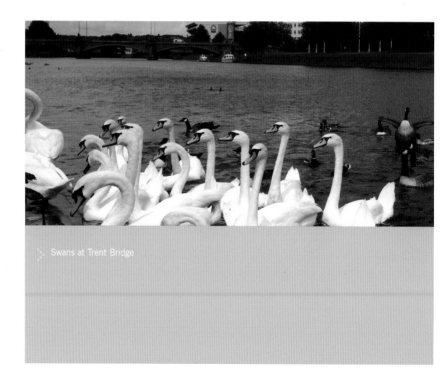

Swans at Trent Bridge

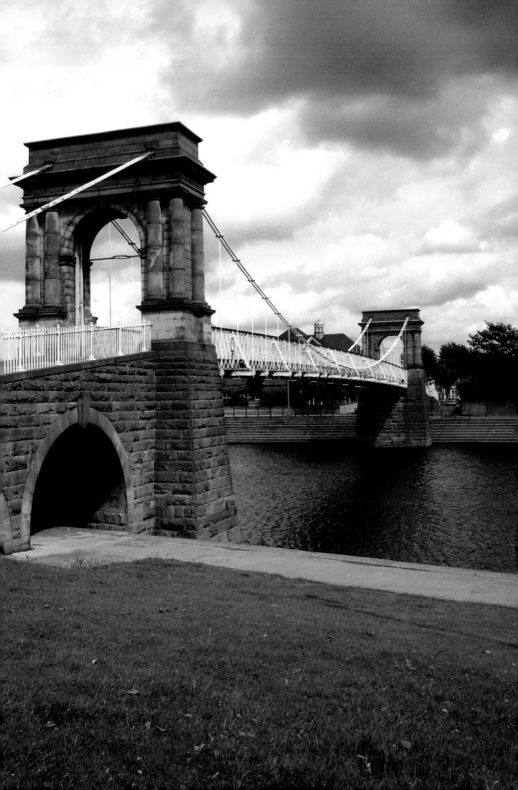

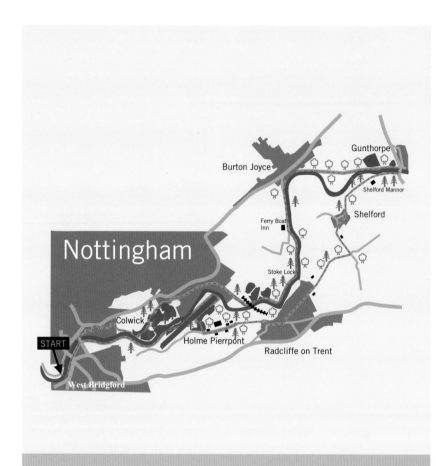

Distance	21 miles, 62% off-road
Time	3.0 hours
Maps	OS Explorer 260 Nottingham

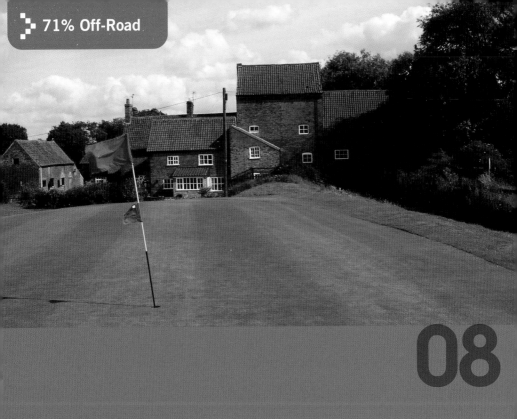

08

SOUTHWELL SEMI-CIRCLE

NOTTINGHAMSHIRE

Route 08

General Information:

Distance	23 miles, 71% off-road
Time	4.0 hours
Maps	OS Explorer 270 Sherwood Forest
	OS Explorer 271 Newark-on-Trent

⇥ SUMMARY

This is a route that takes in a selection of pretty villages and bridleways to the east of Southwell. Rolleston, Upton and Hockerton all have good pubs, and there is a chip shop at Farnsfield. Forget the healthy approach to cycling for once and pig out on this pleasant ride through the English countryside.
The return journey includes the Southwell Trail, which follows a disused railway line. This is a leisurely finish to a route that in winter can be quite a stamina drain.The route can be muddy in places, especially after rain. In wet conditions the grassed sections can become very soft which creates pretty tough cycling. However, on the positive side, there are no steep hills. Also there are frequent breaks on lanes that make you feel you are really shifting after slogging it across fields.

⇥ STARTING POINT

There is free car park at the start of the Southwell Trail. This is situated near the Newcastle Arms public house in Station Road. The OS grid reference is 4706 3544.

⌖ THE ROUTE

Leave the car park and cross the road into Riverside. Take the path off to the left and go down the steps to follow the footpath beside the stream. Turn right at the main road, and after 200yds turn left into Crew Lane. The lane degenerates to a farm track, then a singletrack as it goes over a hill and down past a house at the edge of a sewage works. Kink to the right, go under the power cables and turn right as you emerge by the recycling center. Follow this lane to the main road, avoiding the misplaced rubbish, and then turn left. Follow the road until you come to Fiskerton Station, but take the lane on your left before you get to the railway tracks. Follow the lane over the tracks at Rolleston Station, go over the stream and turn left to use the pedestrian crossing to go back over the railway. On the far side go to the right of the mill and through the farm on your left following the signs for the Trent Valley Way. Enter the golf course and walk to the left to meet the edge of the stream. Go past the golfers bridge, but keep to the right bank and follow this all the way to the corner of the golf links. Just to your right you will find a bridge over the stream. On the far side take the footpath that heads diagonally across the field aiming for the end of the hedge in the distance. Go through the gap in this hedge and keep to the left hand edge of the field you enter. Follow this footpath for two fields before it becomes a firm track that takes you over a stream and up into Upton. At the main road turn left and go past the French Horn pub.

Turn right onto the lane opposite the green and telephone box. Follow this lane for 3/4 mile and then turn left at the main road. Turn right on the signed bridleway that goes beside the farmhouse. After 200yds bear to the left and the going will start to get tough. When you enter the open field turn right and keep to the hedge heading towards the wood. Go through the gate on your right at the end of the field, but continue on your previous direction to go up through the wood. At the top of the rise enter the open field and keep the hedge on your right as you maintain the same direction. Continue on this line to the end of the field, then kink right and left to pick up a much better track that descends towards the tree line in the distance. Go straight through the farm, and over the fence. Kink left and right to pick up the firm track past the barns and then bear left past the new house at the end of the wooded area. At the road turn left and follow it to Hockerton. At the main road turn right, and after 1 mile turn right again onto the lane signed to Winkburn.

As you enter the village take Roewood Lane on your left which is a signed RUPP. Go to the wood ahead of you and circle round it to the right. When the track veers away from the wood, follow the edge of the wood round to the left. At the end of the field go left over the drainage ditch, still following the edge of the wood. Head for the pointed looking corner of the wood ahead of you, where you will find a footbridge over a drainage ditch. Go over the first bridge and turn right to follow a wonderful path within a line of trees. Follow this path in the same direction for 1 1/2 miles, ignoring the Robin Hood Trail which cuts off to the left. The path becomes a firm track as it ascends through the woods. At the road turn right, past the chicken barns, and then after a small wood on your left turn left into a farm lane. After 150yds bear left and go around the left hand side of the wood. The bridleway bears round to the right and then descends steeply with a huge field in front of you. Go to the corner of the wood at the bottom of the hill. The vast open field should now be visible in front of you. If you look slightly to the right you will see a wood about 100 yards away on a slight hill. There is a bridleway that skirts to the left of this wood but it is often ploughed up and difficult to find. Take this direction, and you will soon see the bridleway sign near the wood. After passing the wood you will pick up a farm track that descends to some kennels. The barking will probably have put the willies up you long before you got here, but it is safe enough to go to the right of the buildings. Follow the lane to the industrial estate and turn right when you meet the minor road. Follow this round the left hand bend until it comes to the A617. Turn left and take the first right into Hexgreave Park.

The lane through the park is amazing, but over all to soon. When you come to the T-junction turn right, then first left to take you to Farnsfield. If you want the chip shop or a pub go into the village, otherwise turn left onto the Southwell Trail just before you reach the first line of houses. Follow this easy going trail all the way back to the start in Southwell.

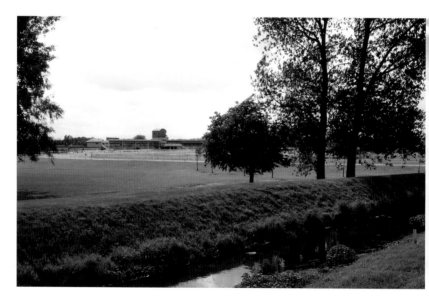

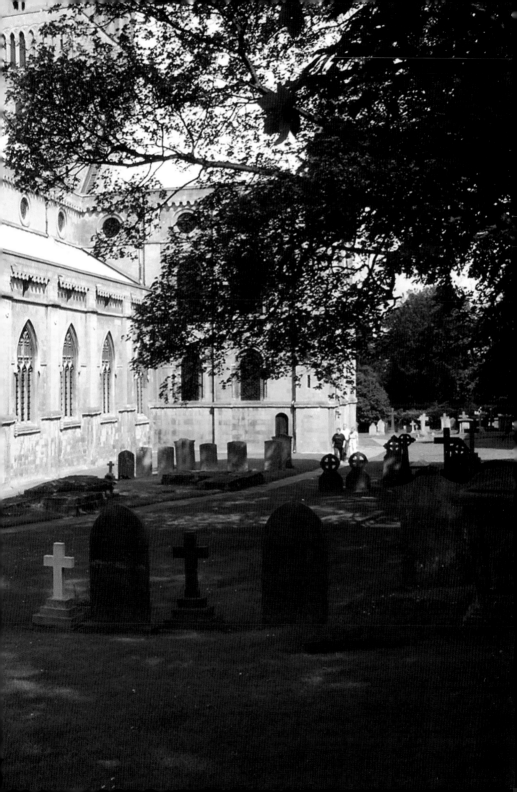

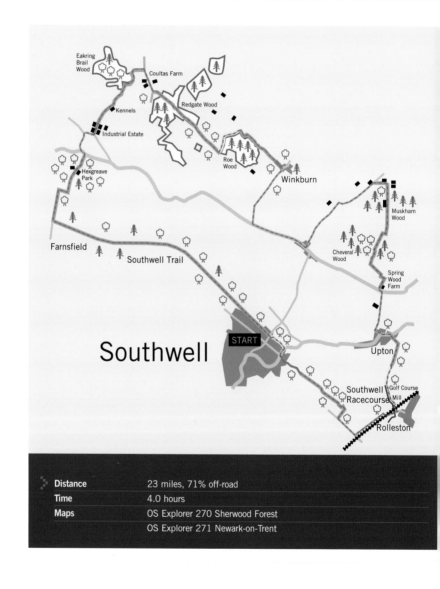

Distance	23 miles, 71% off-road
Time	4.0 hours
Maps	OS Explorer 270 Sherwood Forest
	OS Explorer 271 Newark-on-Trent

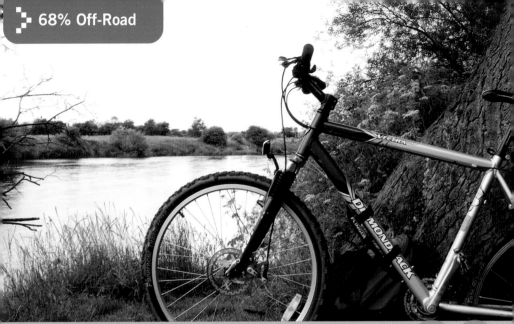

09

TRENT LOCK

NOTTINGHAMSHIRE

Route 09

Distance	25 miles, 68% off-road
Time	4.0 hours
Maps	OS Explorer 260 Nottingham
	OS Explorer 246 Loughborough
	OS Explorer 245 National Forrest

⋗ SUMMARY

This is a route that follows the banks of the river Trent to the south west of Nottingham. It is one of the most pleasant rides going, apart form a short section near a power station where I have had to include some on road cycling to avoid the diabolically dangerous A453 and get to a bridge over the river. The section in the woods below Clifton is stunning, with steep cliffs on one side and the unusually fast flowing Trent on the other. The route back includes a trail through Attenborough Nature Reserve, and a short section beside Nottingham and Beeston Canal. With typical bad luck the route cuts across three OS Explorer maps. However, since 95% of the route is on the Nottingham map you can dispense with the other two if you put faith in my instructions! There is a good pub at Trent Lock, and an excellent café at the marina near Atenborough Nature Reserve.

The route is flat and easy going with good cycling surfaces. However, there are a couple of sections that become very difficult in wet weather and the whole route is best avoided when the Trent is in flood. Trent mud is particularly nasty stuff that sticks to everything, especially a bike. You can increase the bike weight by about 20lb and jam up the brakes easily if you do this route after rain. For this reason it is best tackled in hot dry weather unless you are a complete mountain bike nutter.

A British Waterways Cycle Permit is required for this route.

⋗ STARTING POINT

There is free car parking on the Trent embankment near the suspension bridge. The OS grid reference is 4578 3375.

> THE ROUTE

Cross the suspension bridge and follow the shared use cycle path upstream keeping the river Trent on your right. The path rises to the top of a flood bank and then drops onto a road. When you come to the Ferry pub turn left and follow the road through Wilford to the traffic lights. Don't cross the main road. Just before the lights there is a cycle path on you right which goes round the building on the corner of the junction. Take this past the restaurant and return to the track that runs along besides the river. When you have passed under the arches of Clifton Bridge take the track to you right. This goes over a small stream and then bears left to follow the riverside all the way to Barton in Fabis. It is frequently signposted as the Trent Valley Way, and you can forget about reading route instructions for a while and gawp at the scenery. At a crossroads of paths go straight ahead and follow the bottom of the bank. Don't be tempted to follow the path on your right that goes to the weir and a dead end.

The Trent Valley Way enters Barton in Fabis by a gate leading onto a minor road. When you reach this road turn right into the village and follow it past the church. Take the second right after the church and look for a style beside a farm on your left. Take the track past the farm buildings, and then follow the path that goes diagonally across a field, dropping to a small footbridge at the far corner. Go over the bridge, turn left and follow the path around the pond and the edge of the field. Resume your direction at a small gate to the right of a hedge, and follow the path across the fields to Thrumpton.

Go through the village, past the church and up to the T-junction at Wood Farm. Turn right on the lane and follow it over the hill. Descend towards the power station and turn right at the first T-junction and left at the second, following the signs for Birmingham. This will take you under the A453. At the next T-junction turn right, and follow the signed road towards East Leake. Go under the power lines and continue up the hill until you come to the crossroads with a telephone box at the edge of New Kingston. Turn right, go past the long stone wall of Kingston Hall on your left, and bear right at the green as you enter Kingston on Sour. Go past the church and phone box, under the railway bridge, and then turn left at the T-junction following the signs to Kegworth. Go under the power lines, and bear right over the river Soar. Pass the Anchor Inn and then turn right when you reach long lane, which is clearly signed at the next crossroads. Don't be put off by the restricted access signs; this is a legitimate right of way for cyclists. The lane narrows to about 3m and is ideal for cycling. Watch for rabbits as you go over the A453 and bear to the right. The road then swings left at a right-angled bend near some large rocks and a bridleway joins from the right. Follow the road to the next T-junction and turn right. Follow the lane under the railway bridge, and around the left hand side of Sawley Bridge Marina.

At the main road turn right and go over the River Trent, past the church and then turn right into Lock Lane which is signed to Trent Lock. Follow this lane over the level crossing, round to the right and on until it ends where it meets the river. Go past the car park, around the pub, over the canal bridge, and straight on to follow the towpath under the railway bridge. Avoid following the towpath of the Erewash Canal that goes off to your left. Continue following this path as it rejoins the Trent riverbank. For the next four miles keep the river on you right, passing through Attenborough Nature Reserve to arrive at Beeston Marina. Go past the café and the lock, and onto the road that follows the left side of the canal. After 200yds, where the road bears left, take the bridge to the far bank of the canal and continue towards Nottingham on the wide towpath. After 3/4 mile leave the towpath where the canal bears left and take the cycle track on your right that ascends to join a road. Continue on the cycle track past the playing fields and five-a-side football pitches of the Power League. At the roundabout bear right on the cycle track and go under the flyover to the Park and Ride site. Pass to the left of the car park, and remain on the cycle track as it follows the river all the way back to the start of the route.

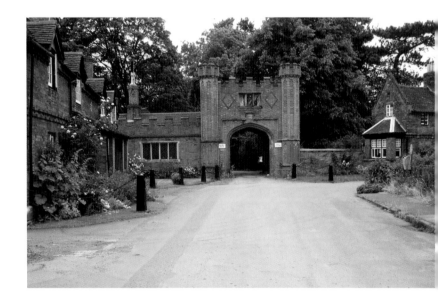

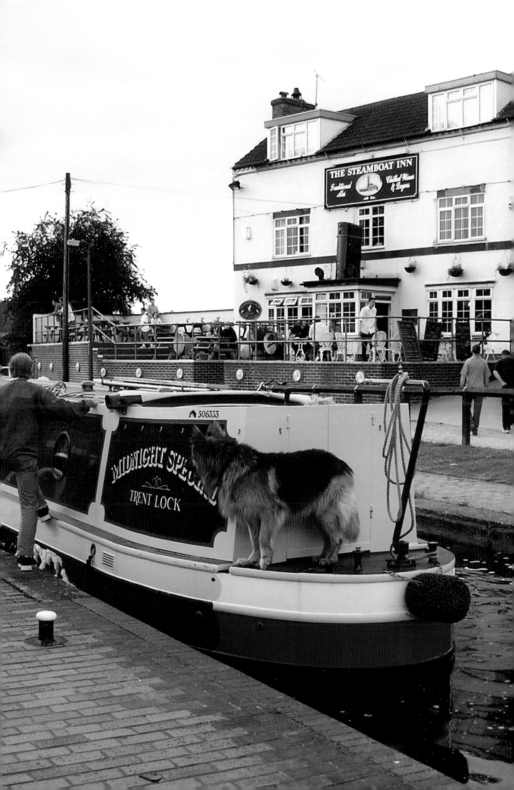

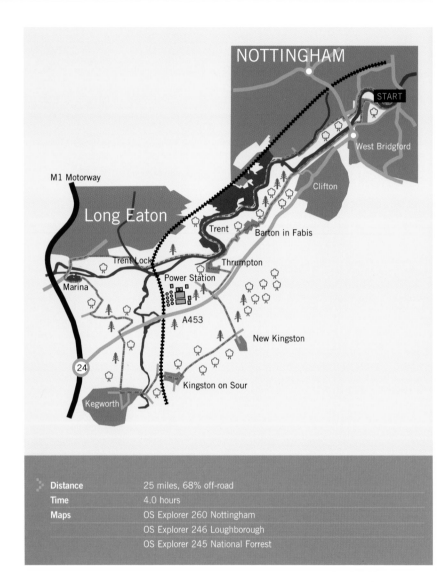

Distance	25 miles, 68% off-road
Time	4.0 hours
Maps	OS Explorer 260 Nottingham
	OS Explorer 246 Loughborough
	OS Explorer 245 National Forrest

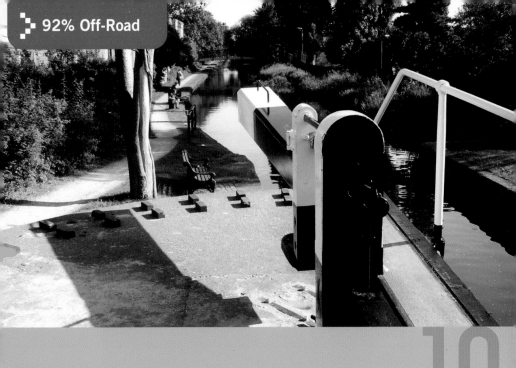

92% Off-Road

TOWPATH CIRCULAR

NOTTINGHAMSHIRE

Route 10

Distance	25.5 miles, 92% off-road
Time	4.0 hours
Maps	OS Explorer 260 Nottingham

❯ SUMMARY

This is a ride that combines the towpaths of the disused Nottingham Canal, the Erewash Canal and the embankment of the River Trent to produce a flat circular route that is full of historic interest. Wildlife is abundant along the whole route, and there are plenty of places for a picnic beside the waters edge.

The route is easy going and the riding surfaces well drained and firm. There are no steep hills, and no technical challenges, other than avoiding riding off the towpath and into the water. This is a route that can be used at any time of the year, but in the summer it is very popular with walkers.

A British Waterways Cycle Permit is required for this route.

❯ STARTING POINT

There is free car parking on the Trent embankment near the suspension bridge. The OS grid reference is 4578 3375.

⯈ THE ROUTE

Cycle along the river Trent embankment heading upstream and away from the suspension bridge. Go past the next bridge on your left and stay on the marked cycle path. Follow this cycle path to the right and go across the road. The route is signed to Lenton. Turn left into the minor road, and after 200yds turn left again to follow the marked cycle lane straight over the main road at the signaled junction. On the far side of the junction turn right immediately into birdcage walk. Follow the cycle route round to the left, where it runs parallel to the stream. At the road turn right, go over the railway bridge, continue over the canal, and after the toucan crossing turn left into Old Church Street. Go through the gap at the end, turn right, and use the toucan ahead of you to get across the main road. On the far side turn left, and proceed for 50yds before turning right to follow the side of the stream again. Do not be tempted to go over the cycle bridge, but follow the cycle signs for Wollaton Park. After 200yds cross to the other side of the stream, and continue to follow the track on the left bank beside the hospital. Go straight over the main road using yet another toucan, and pass the old gatehouse which was once part of Wollaton Park. At this point you are on route six of the national cycle network. Turn left onto the road after the gap, and follow it to the end, leaving route 6 and following the signs for Wollaton Park. Don't take either of the roads on your right, despite all the attractive cycle signs. Go straight over the ring road using the Pelican crossing, turn left, and then right into Wollaton Park. Follow the lane past the golf club entrance, and through the gate that is locked shut after dusk. Go up the track and arc round to the right in front of the hall, past the red telephone box, through the industrial museum yard, and then sharp right as you leave the buildings to descend to lake. Walk through the buildings please because this is a very popular pedestrian area. You should aim for the right hand corner of the lake, and after crossing the bridge take the sandy track on your right that goes up the hill.

Go through the gates and turn right into Parkside, following this road to the T-junction at the end. Turn left into Bramcote Lane, and immediately right into Glenwood Avenue. Turn left at the end of this road, past the school entrance and right into Fernwood crescent. When you come to the main road go straight on into Grangewood Road which is just offset slightly to your right. After 300yds, and just before this road turns sharp left, turn right and immediately left into Latimer Drive. After 100yds leave the road to join the Nottingham Canal Trail on your right. Go under the railway bridge, minding your head, over the main road, and then follow the canal towpath to the garden center. Go to the far side of the center to rejoin the canal, and keep to the towpath on the left bank. Go under the Motorway, and continue until you come to a wide basin where the canal appears to divide. Go round the left hand bend and then just after the right hand bend you will come to a gate. Go through the gate and take the track that descends to your left. Go over the railway line, and turn left when you get to the Erewash Canal. Follow this canal for 7 miles all the way to Trent Lock where you will meet the River Trent.

Turn left on the canal towpath that goes under the railway bridge.Continue following this path as it rejoins the Trent riverbank. For the next four miles keep the river on you right, passing through Attenborough Nature Reserve to arrive at Beeston Marina. Go past the café and the lock, and onto the road that follows the left side of the canal. After 200yds, where the road bears left, take the bridge to the far bank of the canal and continue towards Nottingham on the wide towpath. After 3/4 mile leave the towpath where the canal bears left and take the cycle track on your right that ascends to join a road. Continue on the cycle track past the playing fields and five-a-side football pitches of the Power League. At the roundabout bare right on the cycle track and go under the flyover to the Park and Ride site. Pass to the left of the car park, and remain on the cycle track as it follows the river all the way back to the start of the route.

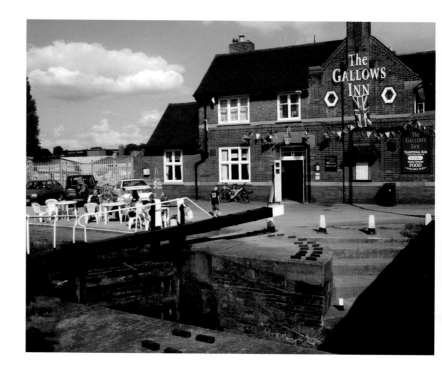

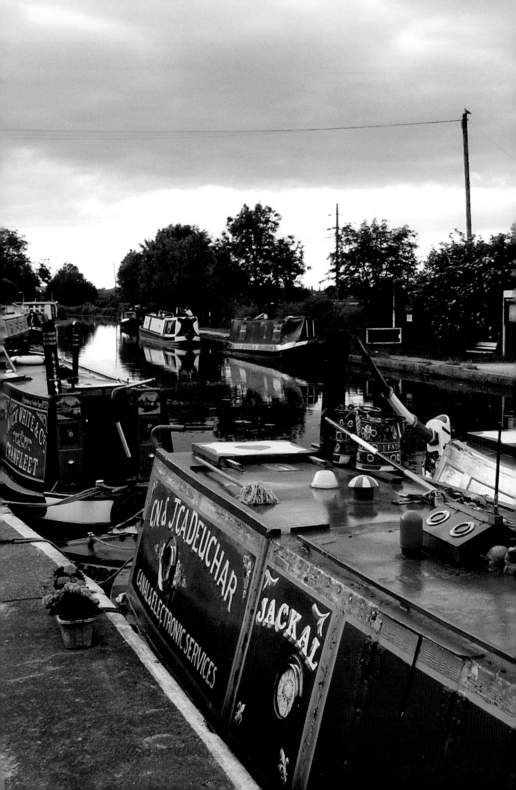

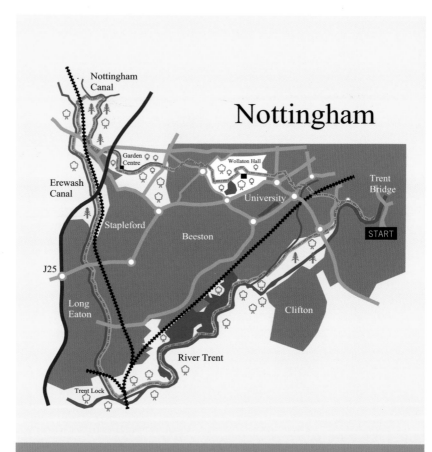

Distance	25.5 miles, 92% off-road
Time	4.0 hours
Maps	OS Explorer 260 Nottingham

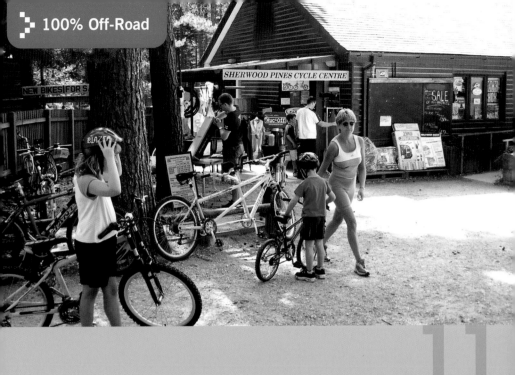

11

SHERWOOD PINES

NOTTINGHAMSHIRE

Route 11

Distance	6 miles, 100% off-road
Time	1.0 hour
Maps	OS Explorer 270 Sherwood Forest

❯ SUMMARY

This is a short simple route that can be extended in any direction by taking detours on route 6 of the National Cycle Network, or routes 3,13, and 14 of this guide. Alternatively, you can just cycle wherever the fancy takes you since this is an area of unspoiled beauty that is criss crossed with tracks that are open to cyclists. There is even a dedicated mountain bike area where you can try a few stunts on some seriously tricky single track trails.

The woods are full of wildlife, especially birds and small mammals. The route is fairly flat and the firm well-drained riding surface can be used at any time of the year.

This is an ideal route for people who are new to mountain biking, but one that should not be overlooked by the experienced riders since it makes such an ideal base from which to start longer off road excursions. I often cycle from here to Clumber Park following route 6 of the National Cycle Network as it winds its way northwards through Sherwood Forrest. There is an excellent café at the start, and one of the most well equipped cycle hire centers I have ever come across in a wood. They can repair just about anything that could go wrong with your bike, and can service forks, brakes and whole bikes.

❯ STARTING POINT

There is pay and display car park at the visitor center which is just off the B6030. The OS grid reference is 4612 3637.

⯈ THE ROUTE

Sling the map in your rucksack and follow the markers through the woods. This is one route that is so well signed that you won't need any guidance from me. At the start and end you will see the green markers for the 3mile route. This is more for family cycling, but you could always opt out and head back for a hot chocolate if you get desperate. However, if you have trouble completing the 6mile route I should immediately pass this guide on to a friend since everything else is a lot harder.

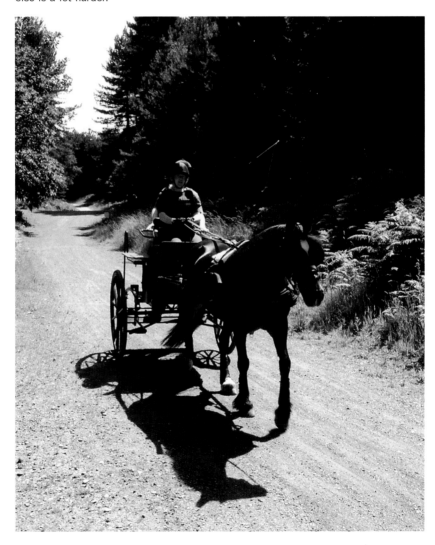

Trail Map:

Route 11

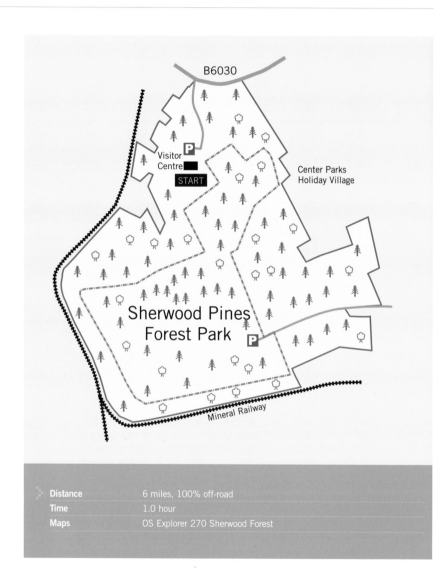

Distance	6 miles, 100% off-road
Time	1.0 hour
Maps	OS Explorer 270 Sherwood Forest

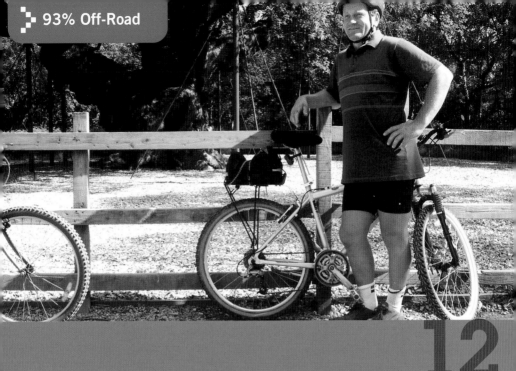

12

SHERWOOD FOREST

NOTTINGHAMSHIRE

Route 12

General Information:

Distance	22.5 miles, 93% off-road
Time	4.0 hours
Maps	OS Explorer 270 Sherwood Forest

⟩ SUMMARY

This is a route that explores the woods of Sherwood Forest with the option of a short walk to visit the legendary Major Oak. You are not guaranteed to see Robin Hood, but you may come across some of the deer .The woods are literally full of wildlife, especially birds and small mammals. This makes the route especially attractive in the summer, though the well-drained sandy soils make it viable even in the wettest conditions. It is hilly in places, but not too demanding because the riding surfaces are fairly firm.

⟩ STARTING POINT

There is pay and display car park at the visitor center which is just off the B6030. The OS grid reference is 4612 3637.

✤ THE ROUTE

Leave the visitor center and cycle down the trail through the woods following the markers for the cycle routes through Sherwood Pines. Turn right at the track, then left up the hill and right again to follow the route all the way to the dedicated off road mountain bike area. At this point the route meets the National Cycle Network that is marked with red squares with the number 6 in the center. Go straight ahead, ignoring the cycle route that ascends the hill on your left. Follow the route 6 signs under the railway bridge, bear right over a road bridge and then pass a golf course on your left. At the junction with the Mansfield cycle route go straight ahead then turn sharp right into Vicar Water Country Park. Pass to the right of the lake, and at the far corner continue following the route 6 markers under the two short tunnels. Pass the colliery on your left and keep going straight on when you meet the lane. Pass the factory units on your right, and when the lane stops go through the gate following the cycle track to the Dog and Duck pub. Go over the cycle crossing into Archway Road. Pass under the first railway bridge and then turn sharp left to pass under the second one. Cycle down to the bridge, over the stream, and then up the hill on the other side. Pass to the left of the arched house and then follow the lane to the main road. On the far side turn sharp right at the large rock, and after 50 yards turn left into the broad fire break following the red sandy track up the hill. After 200 yards turn right by the bench into the first signed bridleway that runs along the edge of the forest. You leave route 6 at this point. At the steel barrier you will come to a major junction of bridleways and footpaths.

If you want to visit the Major Oak take the signed footpath, which is the second turning on your left. Walk down the hill to see this astounding Oak Tree and then turn left to rejoin the bridleway. There are usually a large number of visitors by the tree, and in the summer you can often find an ice cream van.

If you want to give the Major Oak a miss, take the first turning on the left, which is a signed bridleway. Follow the horseshoe trail markers until you meet a steel barrier where you rejoin route 6 and turn right onto a broad sandy track. Follow this track across a wide heath and up the hill to the dense pine forests on your left. As the hill crests you will meet a crossroads of bridleways. Take the track to your left that is signed to Warsop. Go through the pine forests, across the fields and then bear right as the track goes round the sewage works. Go over a railway bridge, down to the lane, and turn left. At the end of the second field, just after Burns Farm, turn left into the signed bridleway. Go under the railway bridge and turn right on the signed bridleway that runs along the edge of the fields. Ignore the bridleway on your right, and go over the railway line again before descending Cherry Grove to the main road in Market Warsop.

Turn left and then take the second right into Oakfield Lane. Go past the houses, the dump, discarded fridges, building rubble and garden rubbish before bearing to the left beside a wood. Turn right at the main road, and after 300 yards turn left onto the signed bridleway that goes down the edge of the wood. Bear to the right, and continue to descend until you come to a crossroads in the bridleways. Turn left onto the very sandy track that eventually bears to the right and descends to the River Maun. When you reach the river turn left and follow the broad track between the lakes and the river. After $3/4$ mile turn right by the caravan site, go over the river and up the hill. Where the track divides bear right, and at the edge of the wood turn left and follow the bridleway past the riding stables. Continue on the lane that descends into Old Clipstone. At the main road turn left until you come to the Dog and Duck pub. At this point turn right and retrace your tracks back to Sherwood Pines visitor center and a mug of hot chocolate.

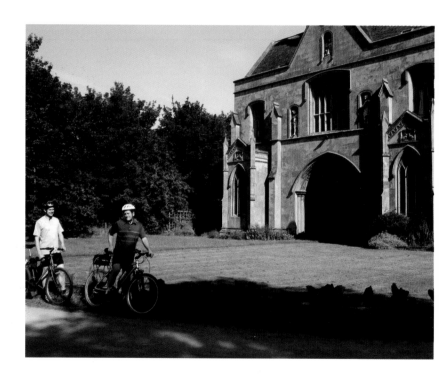

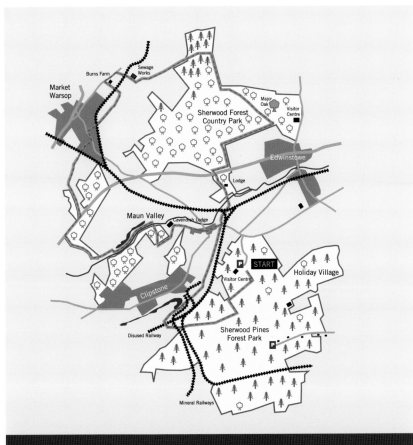

Distance	22.5 miles, 93% off-road
Time	4.0 hours
Maps	OS Explorer 270 Sherwood Forest

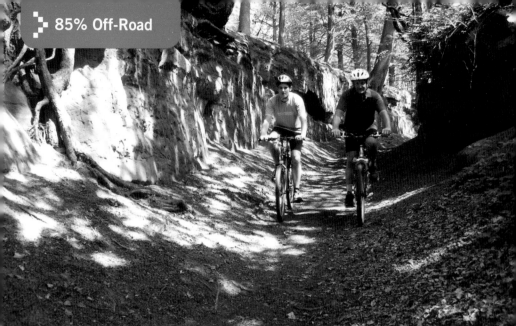

13

CLUMBER PARK

NOTTINGHAMSHIRE

Route 13

CLUMBER PARK

Distance	17 miles, 85% off-road
Time	3.0 hours
Maps	OS Explorer 270 Sherwood Forest

⯈ SUMMARY

This is a very attractive route through parklands and forests. It includes the ancient cave dwellings at Creswell Crags, a ride around the Welbeck estate, and extensive cycling on well defined routes through Clumber Park. It is an area that is full of wildlife, including deer if you are lucky enough to spot them. The route is easy going, with a few rolling hills thrown in just to keep the pulse rate above normal. There is a spectacular descent on Drinking Pit Lane, and the section that follows route 6 of the national cycle network is mountain bike heaven. The route is well drained and the riding surface sound at all times of the year. Route 19 can be tagged on if you still have the stamina for it when you get back to Clumber Park.

⯈ STARTING POINT

There is a parking area in the center of Clumber Park right next to the lake, the cycle hire shop and all the main visitor attractions. Unless you are a National Trust member you will have to pay. However, the hard up or miserly can easily find an alternative place start the circuit by looking at the route map. The most direct approach to the car park is from the A614 down Limetree Avenue. The OS grid reference is 4626 33746.

⋗ THE ROUTE

Leave the car park and head away from the cycle hire shop. Turn right when you come to the lane and follow it up the hill past the thatched cricket pavilion on your right. Ignore the side roads on your right, and continue straight ahead when you come to the crossroads at Limetree Avenue. Go under the arch at Truman's Lodge, continue for 100yds and then turn left onto the track where you see the Robin Hood marker. A bolted log bars the way for vehicles at this point. Go past the log, follow the track through the woods and go straight over when you come to the main road. This is Dinking Pit Lane, which you follow down a spectacular descent through a sandstone cutting. At the gatehouse at the edge of the woods follow the signed bridleway to the left of the cottage, through the gates and into the open fields. Follow the path between the fields as it descends to the woods in the distance. Go over the bridge between the two lakes, then bear to the right and follow the lane past the two private entrances on your left. As the road bears to the right again take the signed bridleway on your left at the edge of an open field. Follow this past the playing field and turn right when you reach the concrete farm track. Go straight ahead at the next track, and straight on again at the lodge to enter a lane which is lined with conifers. Follow this across the main road, past Nursery Lodge and continue all the way to Creswell Crags. You have to dismount to enter the area by the caves.

To continue, pass the visitor center on your left, and turn left at Crag Lodge. Follow the road past the crags and caves on your left. At the A616 turn left to follow the signs for Newark. As the hill crests turn into the pull in and take the signed bridleway that heads off to your left. Go into the trees ahead of you, and bear right where the track divides. Continue to the lane by the houses and go straight over into the lane opposite.

You now have two options depending on whether you want to take the footpath through the Welbeck Estate and look at the dear, or cycle on the minor road to Norton. I have tried to get permission from the Welbeck Estate to allow cycling along their private lanes, but they will only allow the pedestrian right of way.

Option 1 Walking on the lanes through the Welbeck Estate. Having entered the lane, take the first left turn beside the stone wall, go down a steep hill and straight into the village at the bottom. Go past the village notice board and post box, and straight on at the junction. After 50yds bear to the right and go straight over the main road. You are now on the private lanes of the Welbeck estate and only have right of access as a pedestrian. Consequently you will have to push your bike through this beautiful landscape. Continue to the lodge gates and turn sharp right to follow the Robin Hood signs along a deserted lane. Where the lane divides bear left through the gates and continue past the deer park until you come to a lodge. At the lodge bear right on the footpath that leads into Norton and turn left when you come to the main road following the signs to Carburton and Clumber Park.

Option 2 Cycling on the Lane to Norton. The lane leads all the way to Norton. It is a simple case of continuing straight ahead when you come to the wall by the T-junction, and ahead in the same direction at the crossroads. Go straight over the main A 616 and ahead at the T-junction. In Norton turn left and follow the signs to Carburton and Clumber Park.

End of Options 1 and 2. Leave the village of Norton and follow the road round to the right as it passes an isolated lodge beside a private road. Go straight past a second lodge on your right. Leave the road where it bends left and pass to the right of the third lodge. Go up the bridleway through the woods following the Robin Hood signs. When you reach the main road don't cross it, but take the second track on your left which is signed as route 6 of the National Cycle Network. Follow this until you past a lodge before crossing straight over a main road. Continue following route 6 signs until you pass South Lodge, a building that is easy to spot because of the stone dogs on top of the gates. Immediately after the lodge you will come to a signpost with route 6 to the left and a R.U.P.P. to the A614 ahead of you. If you want to double the journey by including route 19 then go straight ahead. To return to the start turn left through the woods and then turn right on the lane which descends to Clumber Bridge. Go over the bridge and turn to the right on the other side, following the bank of the lake all the way to the visitor area and the main car park.

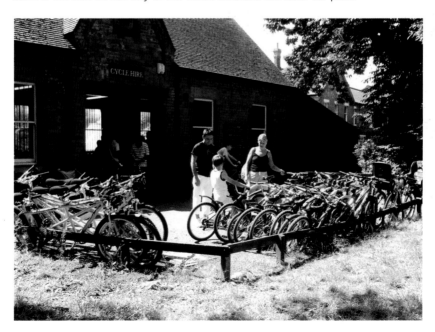

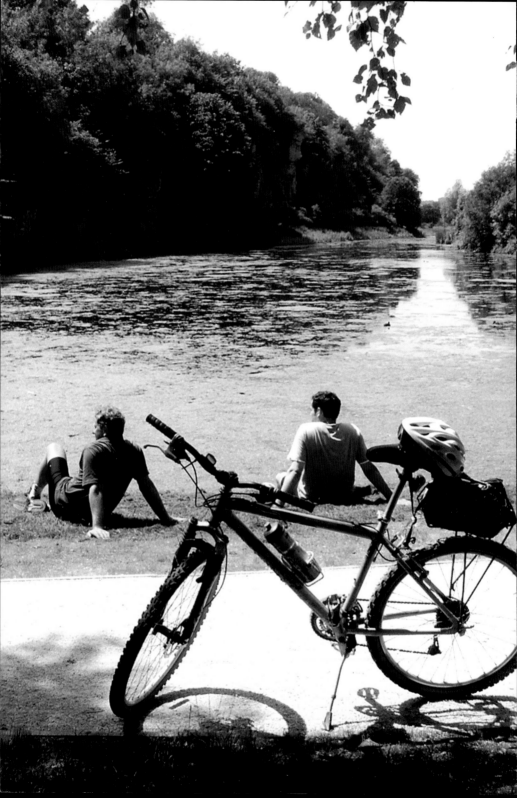

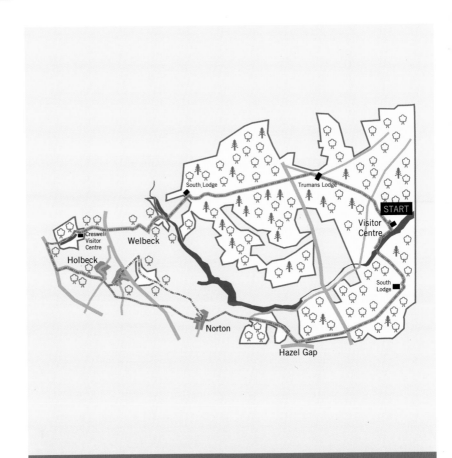

Distance	17 miles, 85% off-road
Time	3.0 hours
Maps	OS Explorer 270 Sherwood Forest

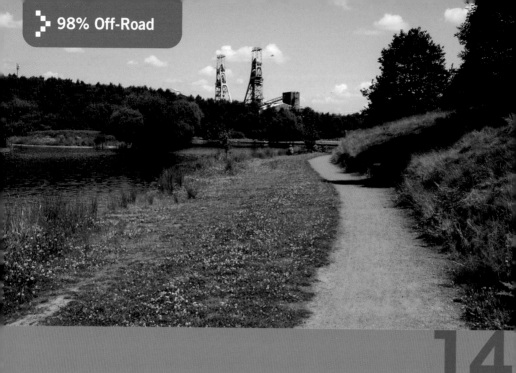

14

SHERWOOD PINES REVISITED

NOTTINGHAMSHIRE

Route 14

General Information:

Distance	14 miles, 98% off-road
Time	2.5 hours
Maps	OS Explorer 270 Sherwood Forest

❯ SUMMARY

This is a route that extends the boundaries of Sherwood Pines Forest Park to explore some of the countryside in the area. It makes an ideal second ride after route 11 if you are just getting started with off road biking. However, I still enjoy cycling in Sherwood Pines even after some seriously hairy rides in the mountains of Switzerland. This is an area where you can ride off road in just about any direction without coming into conflict with traffic. Once you get away from the visitor center it gets surprisingly quiet and if you stay at Centre Parks Holiday Village you have all this on you doorstep.

The woods are literally full of wildlife, especially birds and small mammals. This makes the route especially attractive in the summer, though the well-drained sandy soils make it viable even in the wettest conditions. It is hilly in places, but not too demanding because the riding surfaces are fairly firm.

❯ STARTING POINT

There is pay and display car park at the visitor center which is just off the B6030. The OS grid reference is 4612 3637.

> THE ROUTE

Leave the visitor center and cycle down the trail through the woods following the markers for the cycle routes through Sherwood Pines. Turn right at the track, then left up the hill and right again to follow the route all the way to the specialized off road mountain bike area. At this point the route meets the National Cycle Network that is marked with red squares with the number 6 in the center. Go straight ahead, ignoring the route that ascends the hill on your left. Follow the route 6 signs under the railway bridge, bear right over a road bridge and then pass a golf course on your left. At the junction with the Mansfield cycle route go straight ahead then turn sharp right into Vicar Water Country Park. Pass to the right of the lake, and at the far corner continue following the route 6 markers under the two short tunnels. Pass the colliery on your left and keep going straight on when you meet the lane. Pass the factory units on your right, and when the lane stops go through the gate following the cycle track to the Dog and Duck pub.

Go over the cycle crossing into Archway Road. Pass under the first railway bridge and then turn sharp left to pass under the second one. Cycle down to the bridge, over the stream, and then turn right onto the signed bridleway that runs along the north bank. Go through the wood, and across one open field before turning right and crossing over the stream again. On the south bank turn left and follow the single track until it divides as you enter a large field. Take the route on your right, going away from the stream and up over the railway tracks. Go straight ahead when you meet the first road, and continue in a straight line across the fields with the hedges on your right. At the next road turn left and follow it for 200 yards before turning right at the pedestrian refuge just before the traffic signals. Follow the signed bridleway up the hill and through the wood. When you leave the wood bear to the left and then down the edge of the field to the fence of the holiday village. Turn right and follow the track back towards Sherwood Pines Forest. Turn left when you come to the Woods, and keep the fence of the holiday village on your left as you go up the hill. Go past Blooms Gorse Farm and the riding center on you right and continue until you come to a lane. Turn right and follow the lane down to a car park. Turn left just before the car park and follow the track up the hill. You can now follow the cycle trail markers in the reverse direction all the way back to the visitor center. At the top of the hill, bear right and follow the flat track through the forest until it bears right again and descends to a gated crossing. Go straight on up the hill, past the specialized mountain bike area on your left, and then down the steep hill to rejoin the route that you started on. Follow this back to the start and a well earned drink at the café.

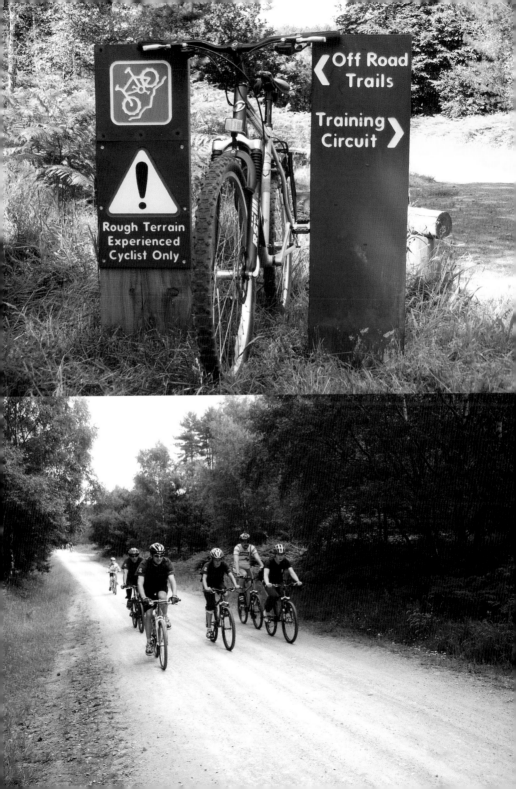

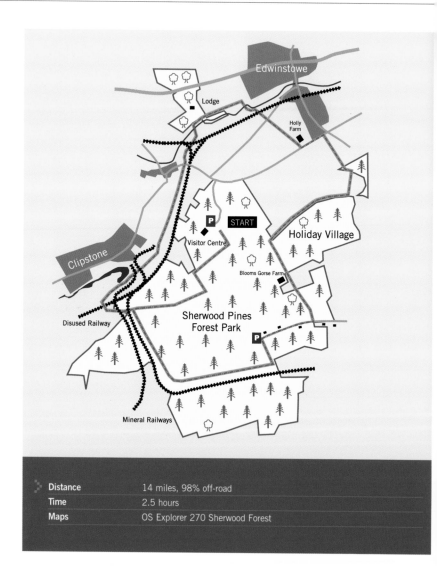

Distance	14 miles, 98% off-road
Time	2.5 hours
Maps	OS Explorer 270 Sherwood Forest

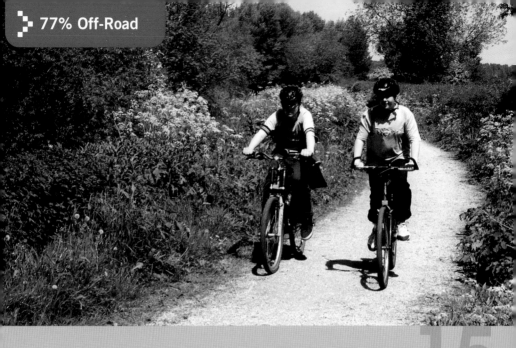

NOTTINGHAM TO LANGAR

NOTTINGHAMSHIRE

Route 15

Distance	40.5 miles, 77% off-road
Time	7.0 hours
Maps	OS Explorer 260 Nottingham

⋗ SUMMARY

This is a fairly lengthy ride that begins with a section along the River Trent. The route then takes you across country to the Vale of Belvoir, followed by a very easy ride back along the towpath of the disused Grantham Canal. It is a mixed bag of cycling on bridleways, tracks and very minor roads. There are some points of interest along the route including Holme Pierrpont, the remains of an old church, Langar Airfield and the wildlife along the disused canal.

The route can be divided into two halves at Cropwell Butler where the disused Grantham Canal, which is used for the return journey, runs very close to the outward bound bridleway as it enters the village.

The route is fairly flat with good firm surfaces that are pleasant to cycle along at any time of the year. There are a few sections that can get muddy after heavy rain, but you are warned to watch out for newly cut sections of hawthorn hedge from autumn to spring. This can be a real problem along the canal towpath near Langar.

⋗ STARTING POINT

There is free car parking on the Trent embankment near the suspension bridge. The OS grid reference is 4578 3375.

❯ THE ROUTE

Start the route by crossing the suspension bridge and turning left to follow the river downstream on the southern bank. Go past County Hall, under Trent Bridge, past Nottingham Forrest Football Club and under Lady Bay Bridge to enter the open fields beyond. Keep to the riverbank until you pass the grassy area in front of the sailing club and enter Holme Pierrpont. Keep following the river past the car park and then join the road that takes you to the start of the white water canoe course. It is well worth the walk along the footpath beside this course since some of the canoeists can handle the rapids with amazing skill. At the end of the rapids go over the bank on your right where you will find the National Water Sports Center lake. Turn left, cycle around the end of the lake, and back on the far side towards the main buildings. Go past the water skiing lake on your left, and when you are one third of the way along the main lake take the track that doubles back up the hill on your left. At the lane beside the gate turn right past the ponds, and follow this over the road humps until you come to a T-junction. Turn Left into Holme Lane and follow this as it degenerates into a muddy track for 300yards. Continue on the lane past Holme farm, under the railway bridge and into Ratcliffe on Trent.

At the main road turn left and cycle past the church. When you reach the shops turn left into Shelford Road and cycle over the railway bridge and past the station. Continue on this road until you leave the village and pass a wood on your left. Descend to the crossroads where Shelford is signed to your left. Don't take this road, but take the unsigned lane on your right that goes up the hill. Pass over the railway bridge, and at the main road go straight across into Henson Lane. This is slightly offset to your left. Go through the bollards and continue up the hill past the gate. In the village go around to the right of the tree and continue in the same direction on Henson Lane. Go straight across the A46 and into Cropwell Butler. Turn sharp right when you come to the first junction and pass the walled green on your left. Turn right when you get to the end of the green and head away from the village. After the last house on the left, and just before the 30mph signs, take the signed bridleway on your left.. This is just a path across the fields to start with, but it soon becomes a wide track that takes you into Cropwell Bishop. Follow the track to the road, keeping the houses on your left. Turn left through the village, past the church and straight ahead to the end of the built up area. Turn right into the signed bridleway and pass to the left of the farm buildings. The track gradually degenerates and swings to the left across the corner of a field. Follow the bridleway signs, and the horses hoof prints, to Home Farm where the track leads into a lane that you follow past the left hand side of a wood. Go straight ahead when you come to a road and follow the footpath to the left of a ruined church. It is worth a short detour around the church remains. Bear to the left, following the footpath down to Colston Bassett. Emerge from the hedge and turn left onto the road. Follow the this road round the right hand bend, and take the first lane on your left after you have cleared the village. This is signed to Langar.

At the T-junction turn right into Langar and then fist left to go up behind the hall. Bear right following the road past the school and then go straight over at the crossroads, following the signs for Barnstone. In the village pass the housing estate on your right, and then turn right into the lane that leads down past the cement works. When you come to the edge of the airfield bear left and then right, following the bridleway signs past Barnstone Lodge. Keep to the edge of the airfield and avoid taking the Bridlepath to the Lodge itself. After 1/4 mile there is a slight kink to the left in the bridleway that occurs just before an open field. If you come to the dead end at this field go back 20yds and follow the horses hoof prints. Continue in the same direction after the kink, following the edges of the fields and bridleway signs all the way to Stathern Lodge. At the lodge conditions improve, and a small lane leads too the canal at Stathern Bridge.

At the canal turn right and follow the towpath all the way to Nottingham. The towpath provides good cycling conditions all the way to Gamston Lings Bar a busy, high speed road on the outskirts of Nottingham. Cross this with caution using the opening in the safety fence just to the right of the end of the canal. On the other side of the road stay on the verge and turn left for 50 yards until you see the sign for the continuation of the canal. Follow this to the right and resume your journey on the left bank. Your next obstacle is a bridge under the A6011 and a gap in the safety fence to get back to the towpath. Here you need to be careful down the steps under the bridge or you will end up in the canal. The road crossing is equally dangerous so leave a big gap in the traffic. The canal towpath gets very narrow for the last half mile and eventually you pop out of a gate near a pelican crossing. Turn right into Rutland Road, go over the canal and turn left at the T-junction. This is also Rutland Road. Follow it to the end and turn left at Trent Boulevard. Just before the signals turn right into Holme Road and pass the playing fields. After passing the adventure play area with a half pipe, turn left to follow the path down to the river. Turn left to proceed upstream under the old railway bridge, past the end of the canal, and under Nottingham Forrest's Trent End. Follow the path that goes down to your right and under Trent Bridge. Continue along the riverside until you reach the suspension bridge and collapse when you cross it to get to the start of the route.

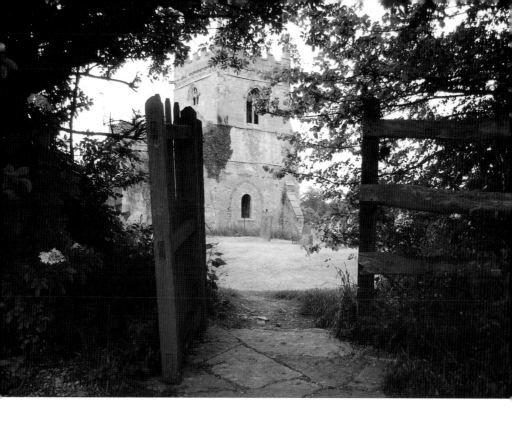

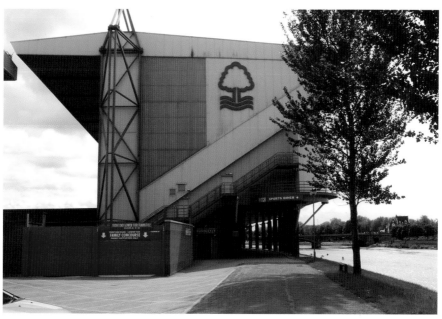

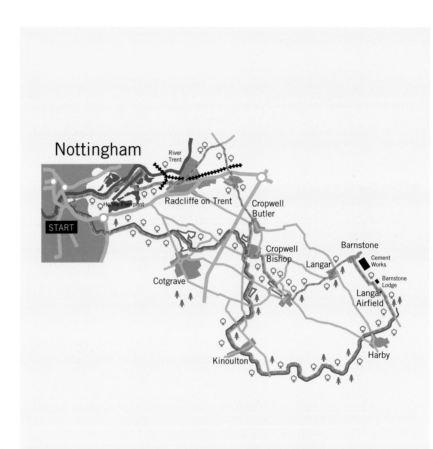

Distance	40.5 miles, 77% off-road
Time	7.0 hours
Maps	OS Explorer 260 Nottingham

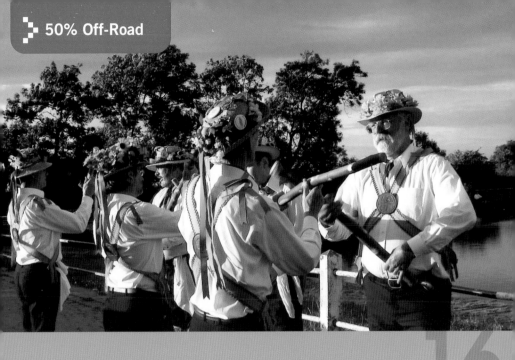

16

HICKLING

NOTTINGHAMSHIRE

Route 16

HICKLING

Distance	17.5 miles, 50% off-road
Time	3.0 hours
Maps	OS Explorer 246 Loughborough

⫸ SUMMARY

This route explores the countryside and villages to the south east of Nottingham. It starts in the village of Hickling right next to a picturesque canal basin. You are advised to get a drink in the Plough before you start the ride, and another when you get back. The route begins with an on road climb that gets you up the escarpment onto a ridge that overlooks the Vale of Belvoir. The route then follows the ridge before descending into Long Clawson. A disused canal towpath is used for the return to Hickling.

There is a mixture of easy cycling on quiet country lanes and very difficult off road sections on ground that is churned up by farm animals and horses. You will get muddy in summer, and diabolically muddy in winter. You are strongly advised to pick a hot sunny day after a prolonged drought for this route. I have tried it on a very wet winters day and ended up in squelchy mud over a foot deep which I defy anyone to cycle through. There are probably a few loony mountain bike riders out there who will rise to this challenge, but it is not for the squeamish and certainly not for beginners.

⫸ STARTING POINT

Park beside the canal basin in Hickling. This is directly opposite "The Plough" public house. The OS grid reference is 4691 3294.

❯ THE ROUTE

Cycle away from the canal with the Plough on your right and the canal basin on your left. Head towards the center of the village and turn right into Bridegate Lane, directly opposite the fancy sign. Follow the road up the hill and enter a farm track on the opposite side of the main road. This is slightly offset to the left, but is clearly marked as a bridleway. Go through Manor farm using the gates, and bear left after passing the buildings. Head downhill to the far corner of the field and turn right when you reach the small stream at the bottom. Do not cross the stream, but follow it towards the railway bridge that is clearly visible from this point. This is one of the boggy sections of the route, and don't say that I haven't warned you. Go under the railway bridge, which can sometimes involve paddling through a foot of water, and bear right to cross a small bridge at the far side of the field. As you ascend the hill keep the hedge on your left, and don't be tempted to switch sides. You will pass a pond on your left as the hill starts to crest. At this point continue in the same direction to the far side of the field. Turn left at the track and follow it past the stables to a crossroads at Top Cottage. Go straight across into the lane on the far side.

Follow the lane past two side roads signed to Dalby and turn left when you come to the T-junction at the main road. After 400 yards turn right to Grimston. In the village follow the road round a left hand bend and after the right hand bend look out for a horseshoe sign in a farm entrance on your left. Go through the gates and across the first field. In the second field keep to the left of the hedge in front of you and follow it down to the bottom right hand corner of the field. Cross the stream and head up to the gate on the right of a farm. You cross a tunneled railway line at this point, which is only just visible in the deep cutting. Go past the farm and follow the track as far as the sharp left hand bend where you will notice a gate, and a path leading away to the right of a wood. Follow the path down to the hollow, veering slightly to the right to find a crossing point over the marshy ground. Then climb up the hill, veering back to the left so that you pass to the left of a house on the crest of the hill. Turn left into the lane, and first right into an excellent farm track that takes you all the way to the pretty village of Wartnaby.

Follow the lane through the village until it bears left and meets a road at a sharp bend. There is a park bench on the grassed island, so you can't miss it. Turn right, and after 300 yards follow the signed bridleway straight across the fields in front of you at a point where the road turns right. The hoof prints are a clear way of telling you the direction, because there are no clear field boundaries, just a grassy strip between the crops. When you enter the road turn right, and then after 200 yards turn diagonally left across a field on a marked bridleway. When you have cut across to the lane on the far side, turn sharp left and proceed to the T-junction. Turn right, and then first left onto the lane signed to Long Clawson. After 600yards turn right into a track beside a transmission mast. Take the left hand gate where the fields divide, and follow the hedge round to your left. At the end of the field go through the gate and enter the lane at a bend. Turn left and then almost immediately turn left on a signed bridleway that goes between the buildings and past the cowshed. This can be very muddy here, and if you can't stand a bit of cow muck follow the road down to Long Clawson. The brave should follow the track down to the gate on the right of a small wood. As you pass the wood, don't be tempted to bomb down the hill on you left. Keep to the high ground with the hedge on your right. Veer round to the left and avoid straying into any of the fields on your right. After 400 yards you will see that the wood to your left rises up the hill, and that there are two yellow poles in front of you. Head to these poles, and descend rapidly into Long Clawson, passing to the left of the windmill. In the village turn right, follow the winding road past the pub, and left into Canal Lane. This is signed to Colston Bassett. After 11/2 miles you will come to a bridge over the disused Grantham Canal. Turn left on the canal towpath and follow it back to the starting point at Hickling.

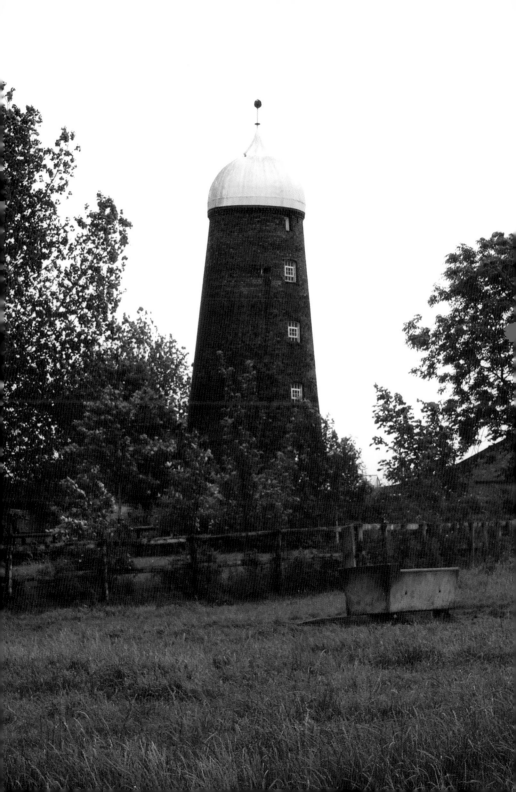

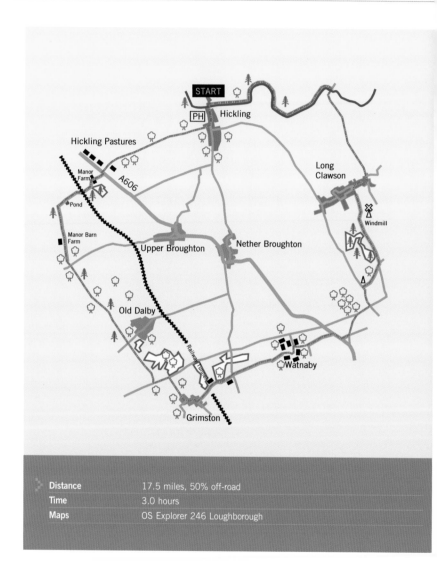

Distance	17.5 miles, 50% off-road
Time	3.0 hours
Maps	OS Explorer 246 Loughborough

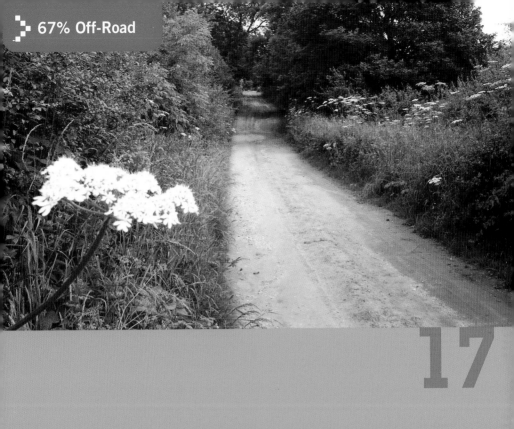

17

BELVOIR CASTLE

NOTTINGHAMSHIRE BORDER

Route 17

General Information:

Distance	11 miles, 67% off-road
Time	2.0 hours
Maps	OS Explorer 260 Nottingham
	OS Explorer 247 Grantham

:> SUMMARY

This is a route that combines a forest bridleway with a disused canal towpath to produce a circuit around Belvoir Castle. The castle is only open in the summer, so if you want to look round it check the opening times. The Red Lion is a good pub to start and finish your ride, but you can also call in for a swift half at the Peacock at Redmile. This is about half way round.

The route is viable at all times of the year, but can be very muddy in the winter and after heavy rain. The canal towpath is just a grassy bank, so it can be very heavy going when wet. It is also lined with hawthorn and you should be well prepared for punctures. This is a particular problem in spring and autumn when the hedges get flailed. There is only one real climb and that is a crippler at the start of the route. After that you get spectacular views across the Vale of Belvoir, a rapid descent to the canal, and an easy ride to the finish.

:> STARTING POINT

Park near the Red Lion Pub in Red Lion Street, Stathern. The OS grid reference is 4773 3311.

⯈ THE ROUTE

From the small green near the Red Lion take Toft's Hill, a small lane that ascends steeply from Stathern. The lane quickly becomes a track and after a long steady climb in low gears you will reach a bridleway called the Jubilee Way that runs along the ridge. Turn left to follow the track through the woods to Beacon Hill, where you will find a memorial that commemorates the early warning system for the Spanish Armada. After the monument, take the signed route to the right and follow it to a lane. Turn left and first right to continue on the Jubilee Way. This dives into a glorious beech forest on a varied single-track bridleway. At the cottage go straight over the lane, and keeping to the left of the field follow the edge of the forrest to the top of the hill. Descend to the road at the edge of the Belvoir Castle Estate, and turn left. Follow this road down the hill to reach the car park near the main castle entrance.

At this point you can continue straight ahead at the T-junction to join route 18 and double your journey. To continue on route 17 turn left on the road signed to Redmile and Bottesford, and descend into the Vale of Belvoir. Go straight ahead at the crossrads, and into Redmile. At the far side of the village turn left at the canal bridge and follow the towpath for four miles. Look out for the church at Plungar, and the remains of the disused railway bridges as you approach Stathern Bridge. Turn left at Stathern Bridge, which is easy to spot, because on the far bank a road runs parallel to the canal. Proceed away from the canal, and turn left at the main road. Go under the railway bridge, and first right on the road signed to Stathern. This will take you back to the center of the village and the start of the route.

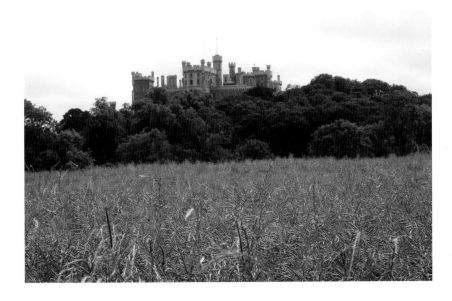

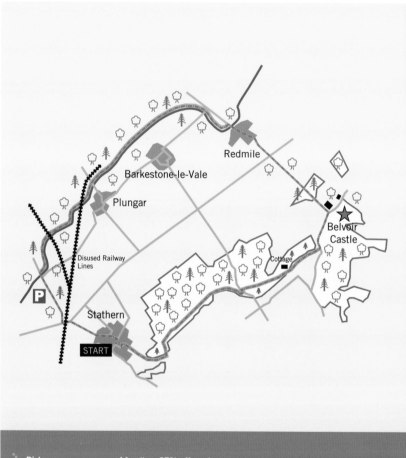

Distance	11 miles, 67% off-road
Time	2.0 hours
Maps	OS Explorer 260 Nottingham
	OS Explorer 247 Grantham

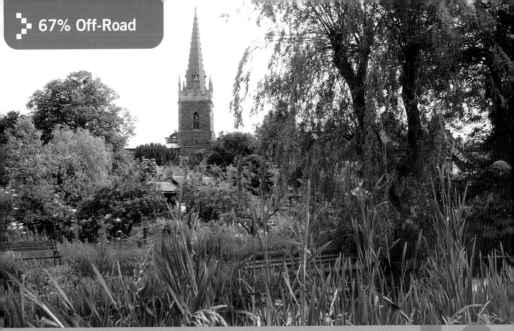

18

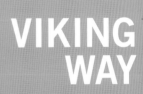

VIKING WAY

NOTTINGHAMSHIRE BORDER

Route 18

General Information:

Distance	13 miles, 67% off-road
Time	2.0 hours
Maps	OS Explorer 247 Grantham
	OS Explorer 260 Nottingham

❯ SUMMARY

This is a short but pleasant route that circles Belvoir Castle. It includes a really picturesque section of the Grantham Canal, and has good pubs at regular intevals. It makes a very good extension to route 18 for those mountain bikers who want to push themselves to a full days ride. The castle is only open in the summer, so if you want to look round it check the opening times.

The route is suitable for all weather conditions, but in the winter the Viking Way and the Grantham Canal can get very muddy. Apart from this, there are only a few hills and the terrain is generally flat.

❯ STARTING POINT

Park your car near the Chequers Pub in Woolsthorpe by Belvoir. The OS grid reference is 4837 3342.

➣ THE ROUTE

Start by cycling through the village, passing the Post Office and Church before ascending under the bridge and up through the wood. At Harston turn left on Denton Lane and after 1/2 mile turn left onto the Viking Way. This is a well signed bridleway which starts after a small wooded area on your left. Follow the track past the cottages, and continue straight on when you come to the lane at Brewer's Grave. The track descends very steeply at one point, and the rutting can be quite a challenge, especially in the wet. When you come to a junction in the bridleway keep to the left and descend steeply to the disused Grantham canal. Turn left and follow the canal to the locks near Woolsthorpe bridge where there is a nice pub on the far bank. Continue along the canal towpath all the way to Redmile where you will see the Peacock pub on the far bank and tables and chairs beckoning you to take yet another swift half. Turn left at the bridge to enter the village and continue on this road. Leave the village, go straight ahead at the crossroads, and continue up the hill to the castle. At the T-junction in Belvoir turn left and follow the road out of the village. It bends to the right, and on the right hand side you will see an isolated clump of trees. At this point leave the road on the signed footpath to Woolsthorpe. After 150yds turn left and follow the path along the line of isolated trees. Enter Woolsthorpe by crossing the bridge and following the lane back to the Post Office.

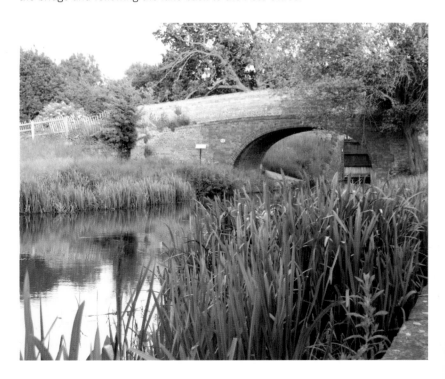

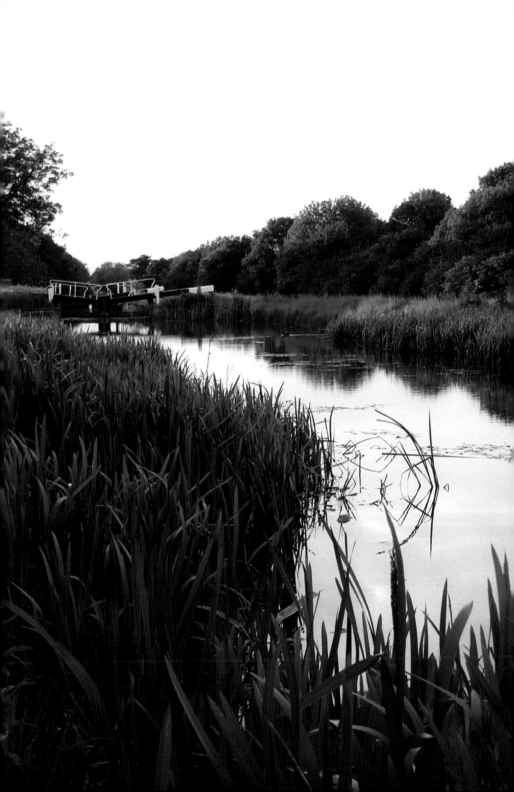

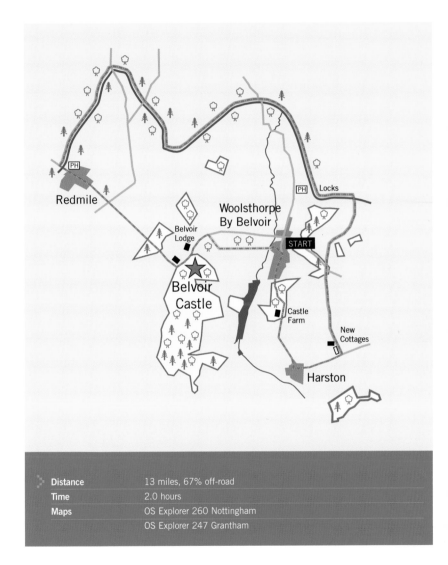

Distance	13 miles, 67% off-road
Time	2.0 hours
Maps	OS Explorer 260 Nottingham
	OS Explorer 247 Grantham

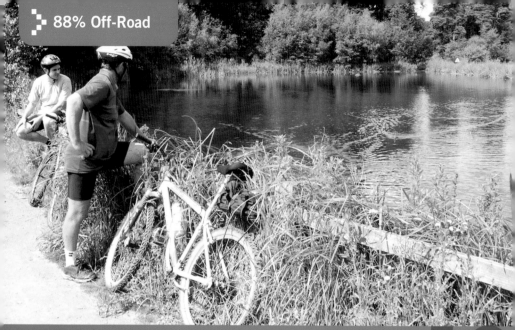

88% Off-Road

19

CLUMBER PARK REVISITED

NOTTINGHAMSHIRE

Route 19

General Information:

Distance	9 miles, 88% off-road
Time	1.5 hours
Maps	OS Explorer 270 Sherwood Forest

:> SUMMARY

This is a route that makes an excellent short ride in its own right, or a breathtaking extension to route 13. It includes some picturesque riding around Clumber Park, and even includes a chance to see the oil wells of Nottinghamshire, though don't expect anything on the scale of Dallas. The route is fairly flat and firm for most of its length so the going is easy. It is also fairly well drained so it can be used at any time of the year. There is a deep ford for the adventurous mountain bikers but wimps can cut this out if they don't want to get wet.

:> STARTING POINT

There is a parking area in the center of Clumber Park right next to the lake, the cycle hire shop and all the main visitor attractions. Unless you are a National Trust member you will have to pay. However, the hard up or miserly can easily find an alternative place start the circuit by looking at the route map. The most direct approach to the car park is from the A614 down Limetree Avenue. The OS grid reference is 4626 33746.

❯ THE ROUTE

Leave the car park and head away from the cycle hire shop. When you meet the lane bear to the left and head down towards the lake. Follow the edge of the lake round to the right and go over Clumber Bridge. On the far side follow the lane up the hill, which is signed to South Lodge. Just before the lodge, which is easy to spot because of the stone dogs on top of the gates, turn left into the woods on the track signed as route 6 of the National Cycle Network.. You will then come to a signpost with route 6 to the right and RUPP to A614 left. Turn left, and after following the RUPP for 1½ miles go straight over the A614 into the road on the far side that is signed to Bothamsall. Pass a small isolated clump of pine trees and then an oil well beside the road. One field on from the oil well turn left onto the signed bridleway beside the hedge. Go straight on under the power lines and up the slight incline to the buildings ahead, one of which turns out to be an old railway carriage. Follow the track down the hill and go straight over the lane. Follow the telegraph poles across the open field on a sandy path that leads to the woods. Enter the woods and continue in the same direction until you come to a large clearing. Head diagonally across this to the far corner and plunge into the ford if you dare. Wimps can take the bridge on the left.

Enter the lane on the far side, and after 100yds turn left following the signed bridleway past the farm. Follow the track beside the telegraph poles that lead you straight into a wood. At the far side of the wood avoid the better track to your right and go straight on under the power lines. Keep the river on your left and the slag heap on your right as you proceed to the main road (A614). Go over the road and enter the woods by the lay-by on the far side. Follow the bridleway to the lane at Hardwick and turn right. Go past the phone box and turn left on the lane opposite the cross. Drop down to the lake and across the causeway. Keep to the left and follow the clearly marked cycle trail all the way back to the cycle hire shop next to the car park. The cycle hire shop will give you free maps if you want to explore some more short rides around Clumber Park.

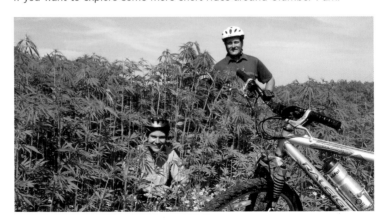

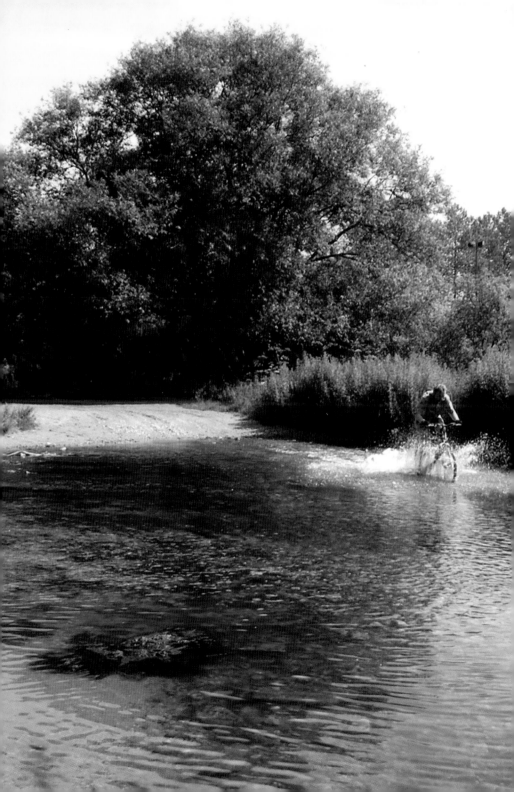

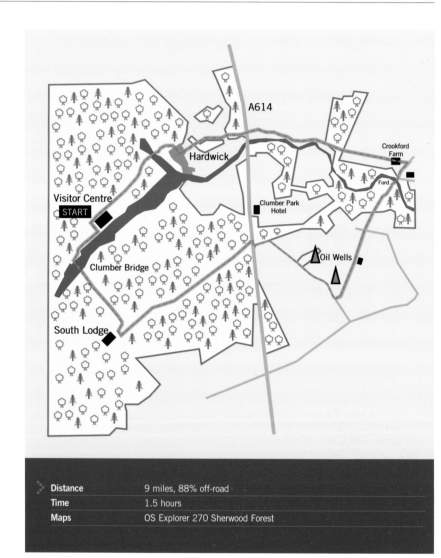

Distance	9 miles, 88% off-road
Time	1.5 hours
Maps	OS Explorer 270 Sherwood Forest

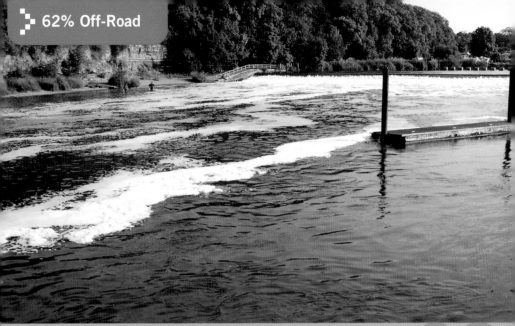

62% Off-Road

20

LOWDHAM, EPPERSTONE AND BLEASBY

NOTTINGHAMSHIRE

Route 20

Distance	18 miles, 62% off-road
Time	3.0 hours
Maps	OS Explorer 270 Sherwood Forest
	OS Explorer 260 Nottingham

⮞ SUMMARY

This is an enjoyable route that combines the wide flood plain of the River Trent and some interesting bridleways that link the villages of Thurgaton, Epperstone and Lowdham. It gives wide open views of the Nottinghamshire countryside and the unspoilt areas that can still be found just a short distance away from the main roads. There is a pub in every village so you can stop as often as you want for a quick half. There is also a tea shop at Bleasby which is popular with both walkers and cyclists.

The route is easy going and there are very few hills. The bridleways are mostly firm, and you can do some fairly fast cycling at any time of the year.

⮞ STARTING POINT

There is payment car park beside the river at Gunthorpe, just off the A6097. The OS grid reference is 4683 3437. Alternatively, you can park in the village itself and cycle down to the riverbank.

⊳ THE ROUTE

Follow the River Trent downstream past the Unicorn Hotel and Gunthorpe Lock. Continue through the open fields sticking fairly closely to the riverbank. When you reach the lane carry straight on past Ferry Farm Park and Restaurant and turn away from the river at the sharp left hand bend. At the T-junction carry straight on into Gonalston lane. Go past the phone box, out of the village, and over a small bridge. Turn right into the signed bridleway when you reach the overhead power lines. At the private drive bear right, and then turn right and first left across the lane, still following the bridleway signs. Keep to the right of the field, following the horses hoof prints. Go straight over the gravel track, though the gate, and then follow the hedge on your right. At the end of the field go over the drainage ditch, and follow the farm track that heads off in the in the same direction. Go through the double gates, and enter the lane to the left of the farm. Follow the lane past the lake and turn left at the crossroads on the road signed to Thurgaton. Go though the village of Bleasby and over the railway level crossing. On the right you will see Manor Farm Tea Shop. This is a good spot for refreshments since you are almost halfway round! Follow the road round the left hand bend and on into Thurgaton.

At the Coach and Horses Pub go straight over the main road into "The Hollies". Go around the double bend keeping the high wall on your left. Go past the church with the square tower and turn right onto the concrete track just before you reach the private road. Continue up the hill past the security cameras, past Hill Farm, and then descend on the track ahead. Go past the airfield and bare right through Bankwood Farm. Continue on the lane past Thurgaton Quarters Farm and then turn left into the wooded bridleway immediately opposite Holly Cottages. Go straight across the open field following the horses hoof prints to the hedge. Bear right and keep the hedge on your left. At the corner of the field turn right and follow the drainage ditch on your left. Cross the ditch when you come to the railway sleepers, and then turn left again to follow the field edge around to a farm track. Go straight ahead towards the farm, and turn left just before you get to it. Follow the bridleway signs to the next farm, and turn right just before you get to this one. The bridleway leaves the farm track and follows the edge of a field towards a wood. When you reach the trees go over the wooden bridge and round to the left. Keep to the side of the wood and follow it round to the left again when you come to the next corner. Follow the horses hoof prints. The bridleway becomes a singletrack path that descends rapidly to a lane. Turn right at the bottom and follow the lane into Epperstone.

When you reach the main road in the center of the village turn left, past the phone box, post office and Cross Keys pub. Leave the village on this road, and when you come to the left hand bend take the bridleway on your right that goes through some trees and over a stream. Pass to the left of the old mill, and at the main road turn immediately left into Epperstone Road. Follow this road through Lowdaham, passing the Old Ship pub. At the Magna Charter pub go straight over the main road into Station Road. Go over the railway crossing, and at the dual carriageway turn left onto the shared cycle and pedestrian path. Follow this to Gunthorpe, and turn left into Main Road. Follow this road through the village until you get back to the starting point by the river

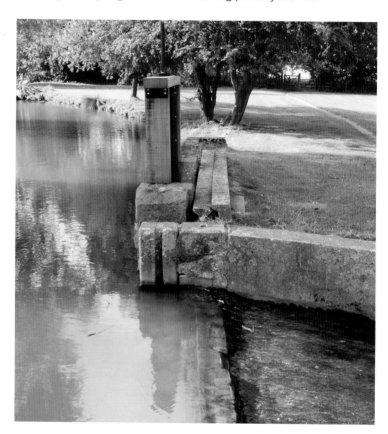

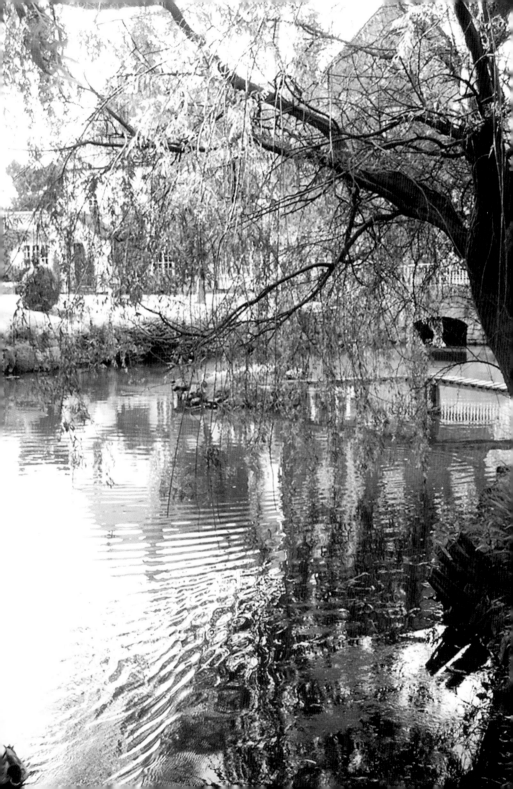

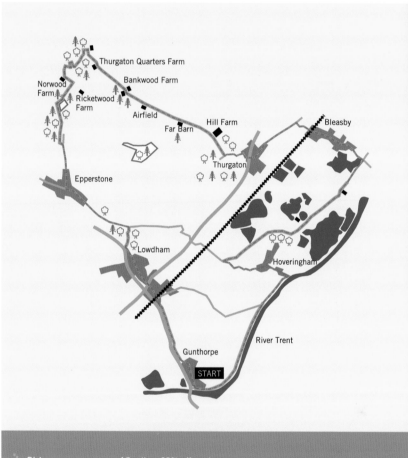

Distance	18 miles, 62% off-road
Time	3.0 hours
Maps	OS Explorer 270 Sherwood Forest
	OS Explorer 260 Nottingham

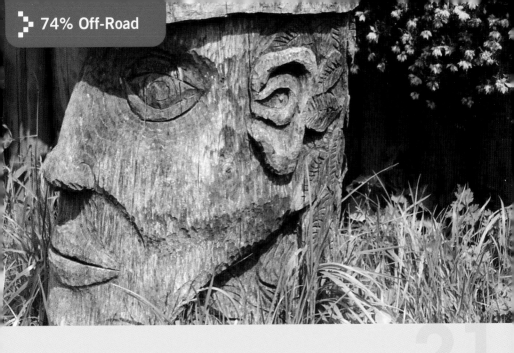

21

TEVERSAL TRAILS

NOTTINGHAMSHIRE

Route 21

Distance	14 miles, 74% off-road
Time	2.5 hours
Maps	OS Explorer 269 Chesterfield

SUMMARY

Given the abundance of disused coalmines, mills and railways, the area around Teversal is surprisingly attractive. This route takes advantage of the Teversal Trails to gain access to some very steep bridleways around Hardwick Hall Country Park. There are stunning views of the Hall from various hilltops, and you can look down on the M1 motorway if you want to remind yourself of the pleasures of cycling. The old mill and pond near Pleasley is a stunning reminder of how impressive some of the industrial development must have looked in the past. Today the chimney and mill buildings stand against a background of thick woodland in a narrow river valley. The area is abundant with woodland birds, especially in the summer.

The route is well drained, and suitable for mountain biking at any time of the year. However, after heavy rain it can get muddy on the single track near Stony Houghton. The grassy hill near Hardwick Hall is a crippler, especially if the going is soft, and there are some other climbs that are quite demanding. The route is varied though, and you get some really easy sections on quiet country lanes. The finale is a flat out return to the visitor center on a disused railway line. Here they serve an excellent cup of coffee and don't care a dam about how mud splattered you are.

STARTING POINT

There is free car parking at Teversall Visitors Centre. The OS grid reference is 4479 3614. The center is a bit difficult to find because it is approached from a residential street. Look out for the signpost on the B6028. The center is clearly marked on the OS map, slightly north of Stanton Hill.

128

⟩ THE ROUTE

Leave the visitor center on the track that passes the old pithead winding gear. Bear left under the railway bridge and then descend steeply to the road. On the far side of the road, and slightly to your left, you will see an entrance to Silverhill Wood. This is more of a reclaimed slagheap than a wood, but this was the state that I found it in when I cycled through. Go through the gate and follow the clearly defined track up the hill past the pond on your right. Where the track divides go round to the right and continue to climb to the crest of the hill.

From here you can see Hardwick Hall in the distance. Continue on the track as it swings round to the left and descends rapidly towards a small lake. Pass to the left of the lake and continue up the hill. When the track levels out turn right, go through the car park, and then turn right into the lane. Go past the coffee shop on your left, if you can resist it, and descend to Stanley. At the junction bear right, following the signs to Hardwick Hall. At the next rise you will see the hall ahead of you. Follow the lane down the hill, past the car park. Stay on this lane through the double bend and avoid the turnings on either side. Just before the motorway bridge turn right into Hardwick Hall Country Park.

Go down the lane with the speed bumps until you come to the car park. Turn right onto the track between the two lakes, and then go straight ahead past the small quarry on your left. Just before the park gates you will see a bridleway sign pointing into the field on your left. Follow this bridleway diagonally up the grassy   field. There is a very steep climb here, which gets even steeper as you go through a small gate and ascend to the road. Go straight over this road and yes, you guessed it, continue to climb up the crest of the ridge until you reach the very top. Go past the stone cottage on your left and onto a track that continues in the same direction for another $1/2$ mile. At the graveyard turn right into the lane and follow it to the T-junction near Rowthorne. Turn right at the junction then first left. Where this road turns left through 90 degrees, continue straight ahead on the farm track that is in reality a footpath. When you reach the bridleway beside the slagheap turn left and proceed to the main road. Cross over it into Green Lane and follow it round the sharp right hand bend. Avoid the temptation to take the bridleway that is situated right at the apex of the bend. When you reach Stony Houghton continue straight ahead into the village. This involves joining the main road for just 20 yards between the two right-angled bends.

Go past the phone box, and where the lane bends round to the left you will find a signed bridleway on your right that follows the edge of a very small stream. This is a superb single track that winds is way through the woods before widening out into a lane as you pass under some power lines. At the end of the track turn sharp right around the electricity sub-station to join the bridleway that goes under the power lines again. Avoid the track that ascends to your left.

Continue straight over the main road and down to the left of the concrete fence. When you reach the coal mining metal fabrication area, keep to the right and pass though the steel gate. At the lane, you can do a quick detour to the left to look at the old mill buildings and the millpond. Watch out for the Canada Geese here because they will nick your sandwiches in an instant. They were rummaging around in my rucksack when I stopped here.

Anyway, returning to the route, you leave the steel fabrication area and turn right onto the lane that goes up the hill. After 20 yards go over the style and take the footpath on your left. This joins another footpath that descends rapidly down some steps and crosses two streams. At the steep bank on the far side climb up to the left until you reach the disused railway line at the top. Turn right, and follow this towards Pleasley. Just before you reach the village the track takes a nosedive down to the stream. Who said railway lines were flat! Turn left and follow the yellow sandy trail with the stream on your right. Go past the pumping station and follow the stream under the main road on a footpath that takes you into Pleasley. Turn right at the road and go up the hill past the Nags Head pub. Continue to climb up the hill, past Newboundmill Lane, and past the miners welfare club. As the road starts to level out you will come to Pit Lane on your left. Take this to the bridleway on your left that is just before the end of the road. This is clearly visible and signed when you get there, but starts unexpectedly, given the new housing on your right. Follow the track until it ascends to a gate with a horse step. Ignore the trail to the right that is signed to the visitor center. Don't worry; you will get there eventually by following the Teversal Trail towards Skegby. This is clearly signed, and descends into a cutting. Continue straight ahead on the trail after it drops down to cross a minor road. When you come to a Y-junction in the disused railway lines, double back on yourself as you turn to the right. Follow this spur of the Teversal trail all the way back to the starting point. Here you can get a well earned cup of tea in the visitor center.

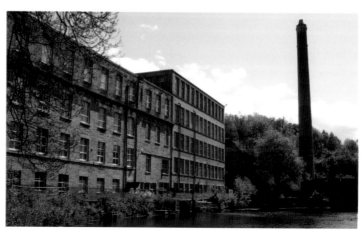

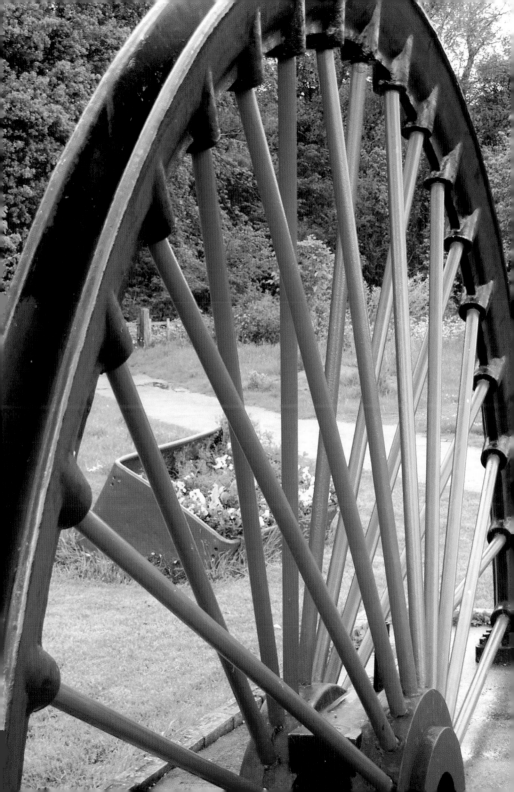

Route 21

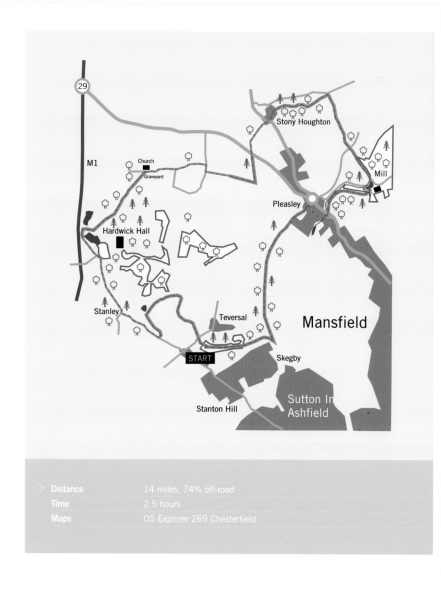

Distance	14 miles, 74% off-road
Time	2.5 hours
Maps	OS Explorer 269 Chesterfield

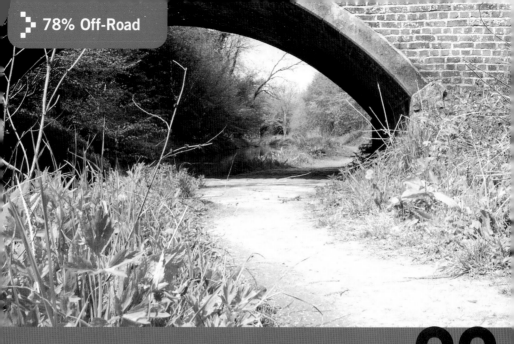

22

WORKSOP WORKOUT

NOTTINGHAMSHIRE

Route 22

General Information:

Distance	28 miles, 78% off-road
Time	4.5 hours
Maps	OS Explorer 270 Sherwood Forest
	OS Explorer 279 Doncaster

⊱ SUMMARY

This route was only included at the last minute because I never dreamt of buying a map with Doncaster on it when publishing a guide for Nottinghamshire. However, after a few days cycling in the area around Worksop I was amazed at how much potential there was for off road cycling. This route begins at Clumber Park and uses route 6 of the National Cycle Network to get to Worksop. A short journey along the Cheterfield Canal then gets you out into the wooded countryside to the north west of the town. The route then does a circular tour to the north of the town and you get back to Worksop using the Chesterfield Canal again.

Route 6, the Chesterfield Canal to the west of Worksop, Carlton Wood, and Hundred Acre Wood are all areas of stunning beauty that are ideal for exploring on a mountain bike. Between these there are some of the fastest off road sections of single track and farm tracks that you will find in the County. The surfaces are firm and well drained and the route is viable at any time of the year. There are a few sections that can get heavy going after rain, but these are well interspersed with well made up tracks. This means that you can always get some relief from the inevitable fatigue that stems from pedaling over boggy fields. The route is hilly in places, and there are a couple of hard climbs. However, they are all manageable and add interest to the ride. You get good downhill payback in a couple of sections where you will need all your skill to keep the speeding bike on the rough farm tracks.

A British Waterways Cycle Permit is required for this route. Obtain one from the address given in the appendix.

⊱ STARTING POINT

There is a parking area in the center of Clumber Park right next to the lake, the cycle hire shop and all the main visitor attractions. Unless you are a National Trust member you will have to pay. However, the hard up or miserly can easily find an alternative place start the circuit by looking at the route map. The most direct approach to the car park is from the A614 down Limetree Avenue. The OS grid reference is 4626 33746.

❯ THE ROUTE

Leave the car park and head away from the cycle hire shop. Turn right when you come to the lane and follow it up the hill past the thatched cricket pavilion on your right. Ignore the side roads on your right, and continue straight ahead when you come to the crossroads at Limetree Avenue. Head towards Truman's Lodge, which has a distinctive arch in the middle, but 200 yards before it turn right onto route 6 of the National Cycle Network. This is clearly marked with red No. 6 signs. Follow these signs all the way to the Chesterfield Canal. Unfortunately the signs keep getting vandalized or stolen, so I will give you a detailed description to help stop you getting lost in Worksop. From near Truman's Lodge take the red stony trail through the forest until you come to a broader track by a stunning signpost. Turn left to take the Inverness direction, which is where you will end up if you don't leave route 6 at some stage. Go straight ahead at the lane, following the signed bridleway to Worksop. Pass to the right of the Golf course, and when you reach the lane turn left. Avoid going straight ahead on the trail through the forest that actually looks like a more natural continuation of route 6. The lane passes through the golf course which is more clearly visible on your left. Go past the large Worksop College building, and just before the 30mph signs turn right and go over the bypass on a narrow bridge. Turn right into Cavendish Road, first left into Edinburgh Road, right at the shops then first left into Shrewsbury Road. Follow Shrewsbury Road down to the crossroads. Go straight across, and down towards the main road at the bottom. Just before the main road turn left onto the shared cycle track and follow this to the Toucan crossing. Use this to go over the main road and then turn right beside the Manton Inn pub. Go over the stream, and then turn left onto the towpath of Chesterfield Canal. After a short distance, a road runs parallel to the towpath. Join this road when you come to the barrier by the bridge.

Go up to the left to meet the main road in Worksop town center. Leave route 6 at this point which heads off to the right. Go straight across the road, bear slightly to the left and through a gitty into the car park. Rejoin the towpath on the south bank of the canal and follow it for about four miles to Thorpe Bridge. It is easy to forget where you are when cycling on towpaths and this is no exception. However, the towpath switches to the north bank at Shireoaks, and later enters a very heavily wooded section. Watch out for the railway line on your right and the fairly sharp bend in the canal. After this point there is a huge open field on your right, which separates the railway line from the canal. The two then converge again, and a very distinctive banked meadow appears on your left. This is easy to spot because it contains some pronounced hillocks, and it is the first break in the wooded southern bank for over a mile. At the next bridge the railway and canal meet and you turn right through the white gates and over the tracks. Go over the drainage ditch and up the steep singletrack through the fields to the top of the hill. Pass the new houses on your left and go straight ahead on the lane to the main road. Turn left to the church, and then right on the road signed to Dinnington. Go over the signals, under the railway bridge and up the steep hill to the top. When you come to the Cutler pub turn right following the signs for the Butterfly House. After the last house on your left, turn left onto the bridleway that descends through the woods. Go straight ahead when you come to the road and after crossing one field turn right at the bridleway sign. Continue straight ahead when a track joins from the left and rapidly descend for a mile all the way down to the road.

Turn left to Gildingwells, and just as you enter the village turn right onto a signed bridleway that bends round to the right behind the buildings. Follow the track towards the woods, but just before you reach them turn right through a gap between two pillars by a large stone. As you look back you will see that you have come through a gap in an old brick wall that was hidden from view by the hedge on the north side. Go down the hill with the wood on your left until you come to a bridleways crossroads sign in the middle of nowhere. At this point turn left and head for the gable end of a building, avoiding the more distinctive track that leads to private property. Go between the two small lakes, pass the to the left of the buildings and continue in the same direction across the first field. In the second field bear left and cut diagonally across it towards the opening into the forest. As you enter the woods keep to the right, following the hoof prints until you come to a crossroads of tracks. Turn right and you will immediately leave the forest on the right hand edge of an open field. Like other forests it is easy to get lost here because of all the tracks that are heavily used by mountain bikers and horse riders. However, if you come to a line of buildings you have gone to far and need backtrack a bit. The right track leads down the side of the field to a gate in a line of trees. Go through the gate, and head towards the church on the far side of the open meadow. When you enter the lane turn right past the church and right again when you come to the main road. Take the first left turn towards Wigthorpe and bear left past the T-junction. At the next T-junction take the more major road to the right and continue on this to the B6045. Turn right and then left onto the signed bridleway that starts at the car park. Follow this enormously wide grassy track all the way to the site of a disused airfield. At this point the track becomes a small lane which you take in a southerly direction across the airfield site, and down through the scattered buildings at Scofton. Follow the lane over the river, and up the hill to the canal. Turn right onto the towpath on the south bank and follow this all the way back to Worksop. The towpath switches to the north bank as you approach the railway bridge. One mile after this bridge the towpath switches back to the southern side of the canal. Here you will find a road bridge beside a lock at the point where you joined the canal at the start of the circuit. Go over the bridge and retrace your route to Clumber Park following the No. 6 signs again.

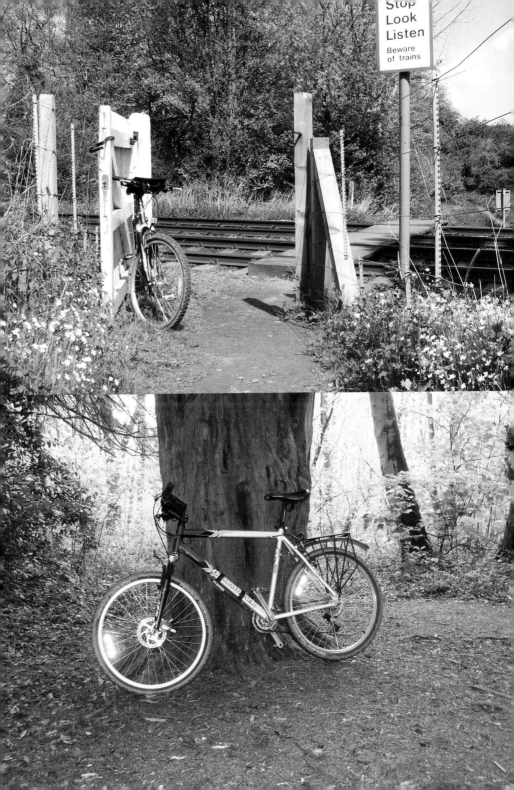

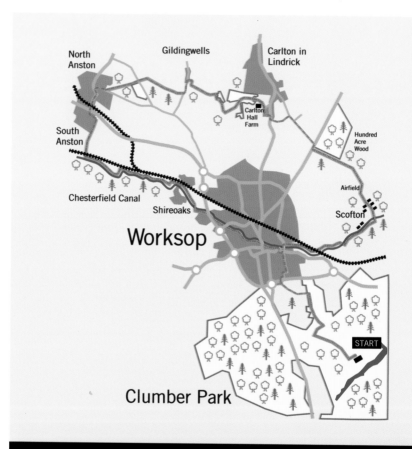

Distance	28 miles, 78% off-road
Time	4.5 hours
Maps	OS Explorer 270 Sherwood Forest
	OS Explorer 279 Doncaster

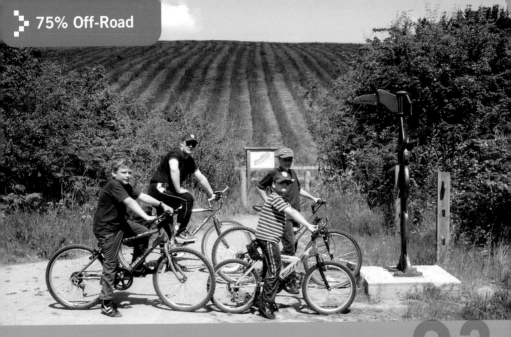

75% Off-Road

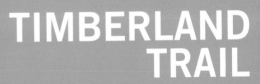

TIMBERLAND TRAIL

NOTTINGHAMSHIRE

Route 23

General Information:

Distance	15 miles, 75% off-road
Time	2.5 hours
Maps	OS Explorer 270 Sherwood Forest

:> SUMMARY

This is a simple linear route that is so well signed that you are unlikely to need a map. It is far from being a mountain bike ride, and is as flat as a pancake. After leaving Sherwood Pines it follows the Timberland Trail to Mansfield and then along the Maun Valley to King's Mill Reservoir. You have to put up with an urban landscape as you pass through Mansfield, and there are quite a few busy road crossings near the town centre. However, there is a very nice pub just after you pass the A60 and the route is quite attractive in places. This is especially true at the start of the ride and in the Maun Valley. I have included an alternative route back for those who want a bit more of a challenge. This leaves the Timberland Trail at Mansfield Brewery and follows the River Maun as far as route 6 of the National Cycle Network. It then uses route 6 to get back to Sherwood Pines. It adds another 5 miles to the route, and includes a few hills to get some pedal pumping action into the ride. It is worth a look at the maps and details for routes 11, 12, and 14 for more information about this area. The café, cycle shop and woods make an excellent mountain bike starting point. If you want more extreme conditions you can always spend an hour in the specialized off road mountain biking area as you pass it. This has some seriously challenging sections.

The route itself is leisurely with good surfaces that make it is suitable at any time of the year, even in heavy rain!

:> STARTING POINT

There is pay and display car park at the visitor center which is just off the B6030. The OS grid reference is 4612 3637.

⇝ THE ROUTE

Leave the visitor center and cycle down the trail through the woods following the markers for the cycle routes through Sherwood Pines. Turn right at the track, then left up the hill and right again to follow the route all the way to the dedicateded off road mountain bike area. At this point the route meets the National Cycle Network that is marked with red squares with the number 6 in the center. Go straight ahead, ignoring the route that ascends the hill on your left. Follow the route 6 signs under the railway bridge, bear right over a road bridge and then pass a golf course on your left. At the junction with the Mansfield cycle route turn left to join the Timberland Trail, which is signed to Mansfield at this point. Follow this along to a roundabout, and go straight ahead into Crown Farm Way. At the next roundabout turn right, and then turn left at the signals and bear left into Pump Hollow Lane. Follow this past the recreation ground and then turn left through the gap in the disused railway line. At the road on the far side turn right and follow this to the main road where you turn right by the garage. After 100 yards, and just before you get to the bottom of the hill, leave the main road on the left to follow the shared footpath that cuts through a wide grassed area. Pass the playing fields on your right and then turn right at the park gates. Bear right at the barrier and go around the far end of the playing fields. Continue straight on when you come to a minor road, and straight on when you reach the main road. Go up the hill to join the course of the disused railway line. At the top of a small rise turn right and then left at the main road. Go down the field on the left and at the next main road turn right and go down the hill to Baums Lane. Turn left and then immediately right onto a path signed to Sutton in Ashfield. You can now follow this signing all the way to King's Mill Reservoir. The path keeps to the left of a park and after 200 yards meets the A60 near the center of Mansfield. Cross the main road and join the River Maun at a basin beside a pub. This is a good spot for a drink. Follow the wooded path on the left bank of the River Maun and go under the viaduct. At the main road go to the far side, and after 100 yards turn right into Bleak Hills Lane which is signed as a public bridleway. Go over the road at the industrial estate following the bridleway signs. Continue in the same direction after you meet the main road by the roundabout. Go over the railway level crossing, and then bear left to the lake. At this point you can simply turn around and go back again or take the alternative route.

The alternative route is shown on the map, but you have to retrace the ride back to Mansfield Brewery before leaving the Timberland Trail. Go back to the pub by the basin, cross the main road, pass to the right of the park and back into Baums Lane. At the main road turn right and then immediately left into Great Central Road. Go past the brewery, under the pipes, and past the Police Station. At the signals turn right and then first left into Newdigate Lane. Follow this traffic calmed road to the mini-roundabout near the church. Turn left down the hill and then after 100 yards turn right into Hibbert Road. At the double mini-roundabout go straight ahead into Barringer Road and follow this past the playing fields and up the hill. At the main road turn right, and after 100 yards take the signed footpath on your left called Stinting Lane. This is a track, rather than a path, and it ascends to a radio mast before descending to a main road. Turn left at this road and follow it down to the bridge over the River Maun. At the signed bridleway just before the Mansfield Woodhouse signs, turn right and follow the left bank of the river. After just over a mile you will come to a crossroads of tracks. Continue in the same direction on the sandy route that keeps about one field away from the river on your right. At the T-junction turn right and descend to the River Maun. When you reach the river turn left and follow the broad track between the lakes and the river. After just under a mile turn right by the caravan site, go over the river and up the hill. Where the track divides bear right, and at the edge of the wood turn left and follow the bridleway past the riding stables. Continue on the lane that descends into Old Clipstone. At the main road turn left until you come to the Dog and Duck pub. At this point turn right and join Route 6 of the National Cycle Network. Follow the route towards the colliery and pass to the left of the black lagoons of coal slurry. Go under the tunnels, and around to the left of the lake. At the far end of the lake bear round to the right until you meet the junction with the Timberland Trail. You can now retrace your tracks back to the Sherwood Pines visitor center and a well earned mug of tea.

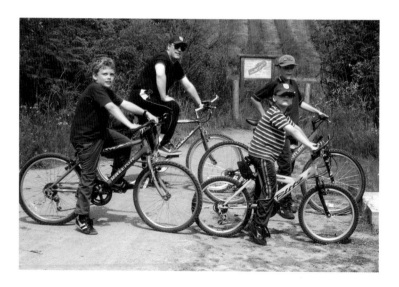

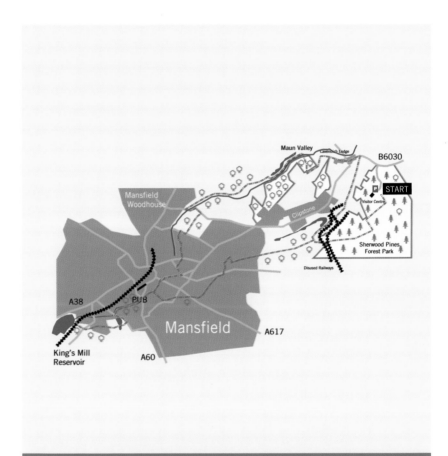

Distance	15 miles, 75% off-road
Time	2.5 hours
Maps	OS Explorer 270 Sherwood Forest

Erewash Canal, Nottingham and Beeston Canal
British Waterways, Trent Lock, Lock Lane, Long Eaton, Notts NG10 2FF

Chesterfield Canal and River Trent
British Waterways, The Kiln, Mather Lane, Newark, Notts NG24 4TT

Useful Addresses and Contacts

Mansfield Tourist Information Centre
Telephone 01623 463770

Rights of Way
Environment Department, Nottinghamshire County Council, Trent Bridge House, Fox Road, West Bridgford, Nottingham NG1 5NT

Nottingham City Council Rights of Way
City Development, Lawrence House, Talbot Street, Nottingham NG1 5NT

The Cycling Officer
Environment Department, Nottinghamshire County Council, Trent Bridge House, Fox Road, West Bridgford, Nottingham NG2 6BJ

The Recreational Routes Officer - for guided cycle rides
Unit 13, Boughton Pumping Station, Boughton, Ollerton, Nottinghamshire NG22 9HQ

Cycling organizations

Sustrans
www.sustrans.org.uk
telephone 0117 9290888

Pedals
www.net-space.co.uk/pedals
telephone 0115 9816206

CTC
www.ctc.org.uk
telephone 0870 8730060

British Cycling Federation
www.britishcycling.org.uk
telephone 0870 8712000